Unlock
Your Muscle
Gene

Other Books by Ori Hofmekler

The Warrior Diet
The Anti-Estrogenic Diet
Maximum Muscle, Minimum Fat

Unlock
Your Muscle
Gene

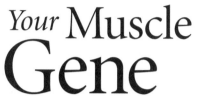

*Trigger the Biological
Mechanisms That
Transform Your Body
and Extend Your Life*

Ori Hofmekler

Foreword by Joseph Mercola, DO

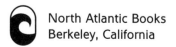

North Atlantic Books
Berkeley, California

Published by
North Atlantic Books
P.O. Box 12327
Berkeley, California 94712

Cover and book design by Suzanne Albertson
Printed in the United States of America

Unlock Your Muscle Gene: Trigger the Biological Mechanisms That Transform Your Body and Extend Your Life is sponsored by the Society for the Study of Native Arts and Sciences, a nonprofit educational corporation whose goals are to develop an educational and cross-cultural perspective linking various scientific, social, and artistic fields; to nurture a holistic view of arts, sciences, humanities, and healing; and to publish and distribute literature on the relationship of mind, body, and nature.

North Atlantic Books' publications are available through most bookstores. For further information, visit our website at www.northatlanticbooks.com or call 800-733-3000.

MEDICAL DISCLAIMER: The following information is intended for general information purposes only. Individuals should always see their health care provider before administering any suggestions made in this book. Any application of the material set forth in the following pages is at the reader's discretion and is his or her sole responsibility.

Library of Congress Cataloging-in-Publication Data

Hofmekler, Ori, 1952–
    Unlock your muscle gene : trigger the biological mechanisms that transform your
    body and extend your life / Ori Hofmekler ; foreword by Joseph Mercola.
        p. cm.
    Summary: "Written in the author's trademark paradigm breaking style, *Unlock Your Muscle Gene* succinctly describes how we can activate the innate mechanisms that help us build muscle, become leaner, stronger, and healthier, and live longer"—Provided by publisher.
    Includes bibliographical references and index.
    ISBN 978-1-58394-309-0 (pbk.)
    1. Physical fitness. 2. Muscles—Physiology. 3. Nutrition. I. Title.
    RA781.H619 2011
    613.7—dc23
                                                                    2011012765

2 3 4 5 6 7 8 9 United 16 15 14 13 12 11

Contents

Foreword

We have an epidemic of chronic degenerative disease in the United States:

- Two out of three people are overweight.
- One in three have diabetes or prediabetes.
- One in two will come down with cancer in their lifetime.
- One in three will experience diminished brain power as they age.

These are tragic statistics, and they are largely related to lifestyle choices that have worsened dramatically as a result of corporate interests that use media to effectively persuade and convince us to choose cheap, nutritionally bankrupt foods that accelerate our path to the above diseases.

The truth is that it simply doesn't have to be that way. The foods you eat have substantial impact on your fitness and weight, and if you are armed with the truth about the way your body works and how food and exercise can positively influence your health, you can eliminate virtually all disease.

The challenge is that these large corporations have enormous resources to invest in marketing strategies that impair your ability to make wise choices. In addition, healthier options are typically not as convenient as processed foods that have been altered with chemicals to provide tasty flavors.

Besides food and nutrition, exercise plays a considerable role in our overall health and fitness.

I have been passionate about exercise for many years and first started exercising in 1968 by running long distances. I continued running for more than forty years, until I realized that it wasn't the best exercise for staying healthy. While running is certainly better than nothing, newer research clearly indicates that running can cause long-term heart damage.

Recent studies show that other exercises, such as high-intensity training and others that Ori Hofmekler promotes in this book, are far superior. Unfortunately, I wasted four decades of my life doing the wrong types of exercise.

The good news for you is that you don't have to make the same mistake made by over 90 percent of those who exercise. Simple cardio is something you want to avoid in exchange for far healthier forms of training, ones advocated by Ori.

Amazing results can occur when you combine the powerful tools of nutrition and exercise to optimize your health. You can induce shocking improvements and changes in your body. The challenge required to achieve this magic, however, is more complex than initially thought. It is not as simple as eating healthy foods and working out.

That is where Ori comes in, providing instructions to help you understand not only the details of the right types of exercise and food, but also the importance of sequencing to make it all work well together.

Like in so many areas of life, you can have the right ingredients, but if you put them in the wrong order, the end result will not be what you are looking or hoping for. Timing truly is far more crucial than most people realize.

Yes, keeping your bones healthy and strong is important, but what many people fail to appreciate is the emerging epidemic of sarcopenia, or low muscle mass, that predisposes one to injury and falls and that increases the risk for fracture.

Ori does a magnificent job of reviewing the new scientific research in this area and condensing it for you in this reader-friendly, easy-to-understand book. The information provided here will give you the practical details you need to maximally leverage your exercise and diet in order to improve your health and longevity and to gain muscle mass that is crucial for you to maintain as you age. It is not any fun to merely survive as you grow older; you have to age gracefully and retain as much function, movement, and strength as you possibly can.

Ori's program will allow you to do just that. *Unlock Your Muscle Gene* breaks new ground in defining the origins of human diet and training, digging into evolutionary biology and anthropology science to identify the authentic criteria upon which humans are destined to eat and exercise.

Ori has refined the concept of manipulating hunger and satiety peptides to boost your metabolism and thyroid while optimizing hormones like testosterone. He does this by helping you understand how you can shift from hunger-promoting foods to satiety foods. This helps train your body to endure hunger as a natural means for weight management and a powerful anti-aging strategy that will help trigger stem-cell activation, reduce telomere shortening, and enhance multiple biochemical pathways that will help decrease the rate at which you age.

Ori played a major role in helping me understand the details of how to accomplish all of this, and for many of you, the information you learn in this book will directly translate into getting leaner and stronger than you have ever been in your life.

Joseph Mercola, DO, founder of Mercola.com

Introduction

Our common approach to fitness has been failing miserably. Most people attempt to get "less fat" or "less unfit" rather than lean and fit. Most aim at getting "less unhealthy" rather than healthy. Perhaps you too have become accustomed to accept failure as the norm. Our society is now getting fatter and sicker than ever in spite of the ever-growing number of dieters and gym members among us. Something is very wrong with our fitness concepts, and most of us aren't even aware of that.

The purpose of this book is to expose the misinformation and fallacies associated with common fitness and present the true, fundamental principles upon which human physical conditioning should be based. Human fitness is not a random collection of exercises, and it isn't about eating less junk food or popping megadoses of vitamins.

Your fitness is a well-defined system. It is rooted in your biology, and it's programmed in your genes. Human fitness is based on specific rules, and you need to know how to follow these rules.

Each of us possesses genes that preserve and develop the muscle, and incredibly, the same genes also extend our lives. Your body has an inherent muscle-building mechanism that can be activated at any age. And there is no need to force the body to do anything that it isn't programmed for.

There is no need for drugs or pills. No need to waste time in prolonged gym classes or boring aerobics sessions. And no need to shove in freaky amounts of protein food all day long.

But to turn on this muscle-building mechanism, you need to know what to do. You need to know what the real triggers of your muscle are, and you need to know how to use them.

So what are these triggers?

What are the facts? And where is the truth?

Facts: Certain nutrition and training protocols have been shown to build muscle, sustain health, and promote longevity, whereas other protocols have been shown to waste muscle, shatter health, and shorten life.

But due to a lack of knowledge, most of us have no clue what to do. We're largely unaware of what we're doing wrong, and we don't even know what we're doing right.

Truth: Cutting through the false fitness theories that are so prevalent today, it's becoming more and more critical for us to know who we really are as a species.

You need to know what triggers your body to thrive, what triggers your muscles to develop, and what causes them to age and degrade.

Unlock Your Muscle Gene takes away the confusion factor. When you know how to use the right triggers, you can unleash innate forces that can literally transform your body to become stronger, leaner, and increasingly healthier.

Life requires you to act. The choice is now in your hands.

PART I

What Triggers Your
Body to Thrive?

Chapter 1

What Triggers Your Body to Thrive?

Your body is equipped with a highly sophisticated metabolic system that is committed to one single mission: keeping you alive—especially during times of adversity. It's amazing how well we're programmed for adversity. The human body is like a stress converter. It turns pain to power.

Hunger and hardship are the real triggers of your body. This may seem surprising, but it's the truth. Challenging your body with these primal triggers is what forces it to adapt and improve.

Accumulating evidence indicates that your body thrives when challenged with nutritional and physical stress. Both hunger and physical hardship have been shown to benefit human survival, and the benefits you get from hunger and hardship seem to be deeply rooted in your biology.

The Pain to Power Principle

Lack of food apparently triggers a survival mechanism that helped early humans endure times of food scarcity. Along similar lines, exercise benefits us by triggering a primal mechanism that enabled early humans to endure extreme physical hardship.

These inherent mechanisms are part of the human survival apparatus. When triggered, they help us by increasing energy efficiency, recycling tissues, improving body composition, and boosting strength and the capacity to resist fatigue and stress. Your survival requires challenge and action. The biological rule is as plain as it is bold:

ACTIVELY SURVIVE OR PASSIVELY DIE

It is now known that the human body evolved to better survive when challenged. Both your brain and muscle develop only when adequately stimulated. Yes, we often need to go through a painful experience to develop a skill. That's how soldiers, athletes, doctors, and musicians become successful. Pain comes with the territory.

Conversely, the lack of mental or physical hardship leads to stagnation and degradation. Indeed, when passive, sedentary, or only moderately challenged, the body begins to waste. The consequences are muscle degradation, excessive fat gain, chronic disease, and a shortened life span. Aging, for instance, is a tissue-wasting process.

Can you block this process? Your body is certainly equipped with the means to counteract aging, but modern lifestyles and fitness systems are not designed for that.

What's Wrong with Your Fitness?

Nowadays, we don't need to hunt, fight, or flee to survive, and we rarely need to endure hunger. Virtually everything that our early ancestors had to struggle for is now readily accessible to us. But this is the core of the problem.

We have been shifting away from our species' original program and from the necessity to actively survive. Typically our bodies are inadequately challenged. And the very stressors that had made our species thrive in the first place don't apply to us today. These days, humans live "safely" like farm animals. And like our livestock, most of us are overfed and overweight.

What's the Solution?

To reclaim your fitness you need to know how to trigger the biological mechanisms that preserve and build your muscles.

Muscle retention is the most critical element of human fitness. Skeletal muscle is the largest energy facility in your body, and it plays key metabolic roles. Besides force production for physical movements, your muscle participates in the regulation of glucose and lipid metabolism and protects you against insulin resistance, obesity, and cardiovascular disease.

Muscle wasting, which can develop from inadequate exercise, aging, or metabolic disorders, leads to the loss of physical capacity and increased risk for chronic disease.

So how do you turn on your muscle-building mechanisms? And how do you rejuvenate your body?

Chapter 2

Turning on Your Muscle-Building Mechanism

Your main muscle-building mechanism is a complex protein called mTOR (mammalian target of rapamycin). mTOR is part of the insulin pathway, and its actions depend on your body's insulin sensitivity. When activated, mTOR signals your muscle to increase protein synthesis and gain size. When mTOR is inhibited, muscle protein synthesis shuts down, resulting in a loss of muscle mass.

It's the ratio between protein synthesis and protein breakdown that dictates whether you build or waste muscle.

There are three primary activators of mTOR in the muscle:

1. Insulin (and insulin-like growth factors)
2. Amino acids
3. Mechano-overload

And there are three main inhibitors of mTOR:

1. Insulin resistance
2. Exercise
3. Fasting

This raises a question: If exercise inhibits mTOR, how does it promote muscle gain? And what about fasting?

The answer is a bit tricky. Even though both exercise and fasting initially inhibit mTOR, they actually stimulate it right after. Let's take a closer look at that.

How Exercise and Fasting Stimulate Muscle Buildup

During exercise, mTOR is inhibited while potentially stimulated, similar to a compressed spring in a box. As soon as your exercise is done, mTOR kicks in with a vengeance. Then, with amino acids nourishment and insulin interference, mTOR acts to boost your muscle protein synthesis to a level that exceeds the rate of protein breakdown.

The result: you earn a positive protein balance and a net muscle gain.

Interestingly, mTOR responds to fasting in a similar way. During fasting, mTOR is inhibited but potentially stimulated so when you eat, it's swiftly reactivated, and your muscle shifts from a catabolic to an anabolic state.

It seems that the same mechanisms that inhibit protein synthesis in your muscle during exercise and fasting contribute to the stimulation of muscle protein anabolism right after.

But there is something else about exercise and fasting. When combined, they activate a mechanism that regenerates new muscle and brain cells.

The Mechanism That Regenerates New Muscle and Brain Cells

Scientists are now finding evidence that fasting and exercise activate genes that encode growth factors in the brain and muscle to convert brain stem cells and muscle satellite cells into new neurons and muscle cells, respectively.

This amazing rejuvenation mechanism seems to respond best to the combination of fasting and exercise. Technically, it's triggered by lack of food, muscle injury, and protein breakdown (such as that caused by intense exercise and fasting).

Unlike mTOR, however, this rejuvenation mechanism isn't primarily about tissue buildup, but rather about tissue repair. It recycles old, damaged, and broken cells into new cells and thereby protects against injury and aging.

We'll take a closer look at this rejuvenation mechanism later on, but for now let's continue with mTOR and its anabolic actions after exercise.

The period right after exercise is particularly important. This is the time when the muscle is most ready to assimilate nutrients and protein. It's called "the window of opportunity," and for a good reason.

The Window of Opportunity

As noted, mTOR is highly responsive to insulin, and to IGF-1 (insulin-like growth factor-1) in particular. IGF-1 is the most potent growth factor in your muscle. Its production is stimulated by intense exercise, but it needs insulin interference to finalize its actions. All this comes into play during the recovery period after exercise.

When you eat a recovery meal right after exercise, insulin acts to potentiate IGF-1, which is already at peak level. That's the ideal time to feed your muscle and promote muscle gain—hence, the window of opportunity.

Let's take a closer look at the physical and nutritional triggers of your muscle mTOR.

The Physical Triggers of Your Muscle mTOR

Researchers have found that the main physical trigger for your muscle mTOR is mechano-overload. Mechano-overload is the impact you get from intense strength, speed, and explosive drills. In technical terms, mechano-overload triggers the release of a cellular compound called phosphatidic acid, which turns on your muscle mTOR to increase protein synthesis in the myofibrils.

In addition to activation of mTOR, mechano-overload triggers genes encoding growth factors and myogenic regulatory factors (MRFs), which turn on satellite cells to commit and differentiate into new muscle cells.

Note that moderate exercise and aerobics can't do that. They lack the intensity needed to yield this anabolic impact. Aerobic training affects mainly the mitochondria (the cellular energy facility) but hardly affects the myofibrils. Even though aerobics yields some cardiovascular benefits, it fails to build muscle mass.

Quite often, chronic, prolonged aerobics drills can actually give your muscle the wrong signal and lead to loss of muscle size and diminished strength.

Is Aerobics Bad for You?

Researchers in the area of muscle biology and aging have found growing evidence that prolonged aerobics training increases the risk of oxidative damage in your muscle. This type of training causes an overwhelming accumulation of free radicals, which beyond a certain threshold will cause oxidative damage in your muscle fibers and mitochondria. This risk of oxidative damage becomes increasingly higher as you get older.

In comparison, intense exercise protocols that are inherently short have been shown to minimize this risk.

In order to get desirable results, the physical triggers must be incorporated with nutritional triggers. Let's see what kind of nutritional triggers are needed.

The Nutritional Triggers of Your Muscle mTOR

The main nutritional triggers of your muscle mTOR are essential amino acids, particularly the amino acid leucine. Studies reveal that intravenous administration of amino acids increases the rate of muscle protein synthesis after exercise and simultaneously lowers the rate of muscle protein breakdown.

Dietary protein seems to be the primary factor in muscle nourishment. Researchers worldwide believe that the diet protocol that benefits human fitness most is the high-protein, low-carbohydrate diet. Recent studies have reported substantial benefits of the high-protein, low-carbohydrate diet on muscle conditioning and weight loss.

A key element in this diet regimen appears to be the high intake of the amino acid leucine, which is part of the branched-chain amino acids, or BCAAs (leucine, isoleucine, and valine). Along with the stimulation of muscle protein synthesis, leucine has been shown to modulate insulin and blood sugar. But to further understand how leucine regulates muscle buildup, we need to take a closer look at leucine's actions.

Leucine and Muscle Buildup

Unlike other amino acids, which serve mainly as building blocks for muscle protein, leucine has an additional role: it signals your muscle mTOR to increase protein synthesis. Incredibly, leucine has been shown to stimulate muscle protein synthesis even during times of food restriction or after prolonged physical hardship.

It's the sheer increase in circulating leucine concentration that triggers the mTOR in your muscle.

On the cellular level, leucine stimulates phosphorylation of an inhibitory protein, 4E-BP1 (4E-binding protein 1). The removal of this inhibitory protein activates initiation factors to increase muscle protein synthesis.

Researchers believe that leucine's unique role in the regulation of muscle protein synthesis is consistent with the retention of lean body mass seen with high-protein diets during weight loss.

So what's the best food source of leucine?

The highest food concentrations of leucine and BCAAs are found in dairy products, particularly quality cheese and whey protein. And even though leucine is relatively abundant in our food supply, it is often wasted as an energy substrate or used as a building block rather than an anabolic agent. This means that to establish the right anabolic environment, you should try to increase leucine consumption beyond maintenance requirements.

But beware that only *food-based* leucine can benefit the muscle without side effects. Intravenous administration of free-form amino acids (including leucine) has been shown to cause severe hyperglycemic reactions and insulin resistance. When free-form amino acids are artificially administrated, they rapidly enter the circulation while disrupting insulin function and impairing the body's glycemic control. This proves again that we're programmed to benefit only from whole-food nutrition.

How Much Leucine Do You Need to Consume to Get Results?

Based on nitrogen-balance measurements, the requirement for leucine to maintain body protein is 1 to 3 g daily. To optimize its anabolic pathway, it has been estimated that leucine requirement should be about 8 to 16 g daily (roughly 500–1,500 g protein food intake from the typical diet as compared to only 100 g whey protein).

The chart below presents leucine content in common foods.

Leucine Content in Food / per 100 g

Whey Protein Concentrate	8.0 g
Raw cheddar cheese	3.6 g
Lean beef	1.7 g
Salmon	1.6 g
Almonds	1.5 g
Chicken	1.4 g
Chickpeas	1.4 g
Egg yolk	1.4 g
Raw eggs	1.0 g
Sheep's milk	0.6 g
Pork	0.4 g
Cow's milk	0.3 g

This means that to get the minimum 8 g of leucine required for anabolic purposes, you need to consume the following amount of foods:

• A pound of lean beef
• A pound and a half of chicken
• Three pounds of pork

- Over a pound and a half of whole eggs (sixteen eggs)
- Over a pound of almonds (over 3,000 calories)
- Half a pound of raw cheddar cheese

Remarkably, you get the same amount of leucine from only 3.5 oz of whey protein.

You can see how whey-protein supplements can effectively allow you to get the minimum leucine required for muscle gain without taking in massive amounts of food and calories. You can also notice the great anabolic potential of lacto-vegetarian proteins such as beans, eggs, and cheese.

Note that the anabolic impact of leucine is proportional to its availability and is dependent on its circulating levels. This means that the more leucine you consume from food, the greater the anabolic impact.

Now that we know what triggers your muscle mTOR, let's see what disrupts it.

What Disrupts Your Muscle mTOR?

Since mTOR is part of the insulin pathway, it can be utterly disrupted by insulin resistance. That's why diabetes is typically associated with muscle wasting. And that's why high-glycemic diets and their insulin-shattering effects are potentially detrimental to muscle development.

Other disruptors of mTOR include nutritional deficiencies and accumulated oxidative stress such as that due to injury, overtraining, or muscle inflammatory disease.

Caffeine is another mTOR inhibitor, but caffeine isn't really bad for your muscle. It actually inhibits mTOR in a manner similar to exercise, meaning you can have your coffee before or during training, but not right after. This will allow a complete, uncompromised activation of the mTOR during the recovery period following exercise.

Next we'll take a look at another important factor that dictates whether you gain or lose muscle mass: the glycemic factor.

Chapter 3

The Glycemic Factor

The triggering of your muscle mTOR requires a healthy insulin system. Any impairment in your insulin activity will shatter your muscle mTOR and jeopardize your chance to gain muscle mass. The opposite is also true: anything that improves your insulin activity will help promote muscle buildup.

The glycemic factor seems to be a key determinant in muscle conditioning. It is the factor that dictates the fate of your insulin and your muscle.

The food that has been shown to be the most complementary to your insulin is dietary protein. Studies have reported that dietary protein has a beneficial stabilizing effect on your body's glycemic control. Furthermore, protein has been shown to serve as the ideal fuel during times of fasting and intense physical hardship, as it prevents hypoglycemia and maintains energy homeostasis.

Protein: Your Ideal Fuel during Intense Hardship

Protein can serve as the ideal muscle fuel during intense exercise. But your body uses only certain amino acids for that purpose: the branched-chain amino acids (BCAAs).

A large percentage of dietary amino acids is oxidized and wasted even before reaching the circulatory system. The exception to this pattern are the BCAAs; over 80 percent of dietary content of leucine, valine, and isoleucine reaches circulation.

It seems that the body spares these amino acids for one purpose: muscle fueling.

The Alanine-Glucose Cycle: Your Most Efficient Muscle-Fueling Mechanism

BCAAs reach the muscle directly to serve as emergency fuel. They contribute carbon to glucose synthesis via a process called the alanine-glucose cycle. This process converts BCAA into alanine and glutamine, which then serve as carbon donors to the production of glucose.

And all this without spiking insulin.

What's special about the alanine-glucose cycle is that it allows you to fuel your muscle and burn fat at the same time.

The alanine-glucose cycle accounts for 40 percent of gluconeogenesis (endogenous glucose production) during prolonged exercise. The rest of the glucose comes from glycogen breakdown.

Gluconeogenesis occurs mainly in the liver and grants a perfect supply of glucose to your muscle when no other fuel is available. This fueling mechanism is so efficient that it persistently keeps blood sugar from spiking or plummeting.

Gluconeogenesis is the only fueling mechanism that yields perfect glycemic control. It releases to your muscles the exact amount of glucose needed during times of intense physical or nutritional stress. That makes it the ideal fueling mechanism for athletes engaged in nonaerobic drills such as weight lifting, boxing, or grappling. Amino acids seem to be the ideal fuel to prevent "hitting the wall."

It's plausible that we evolved to possess this perfect protein-fueling mechanism during primordial times, when humans were engaged in extreme physical hardship while being on a frugal diet that was primarily low-glycemic foods, devoid of grains and sugar.

In fact, this fueling mechanism benefits us only when we're deprived of dietary carbohydrates.

High-carb meals shut down this awesome fueling mechanism, and your body shifts instead to the less-effective carbohydrate fuel.

Is Carbohydrate Fuel Bad for You?

Carbohydrate fuel is like a double-edged sword. Complex carbohydrates are a viable fuel choice for endurance training. Endurance athletes such as long-distance runners have used them for glycogen loading.

Nevertheless, there is growing evidence that the human body has not evolved to do well on a high-carbohydrate diet. In addition, as we age, we tend to further lose our tolerance to carbohydrate foods and their glycemic load.

Under certain conditions carbohydrates may act to prohibit muscle development. A recent study revealed that adding simple carbohydrates to protein supplements negated the anabolic effect of the protein and blunted muscle protein synthesis in a group of healthy people over the age of sixty.

One of the major problems with today's fitness practices is the ignorance toward muscle fueling. We have been shifting away from the primal low-glycemic fuel (protein and fat) into the high-glycemic fuel (refined carbohydrates). Again, we pay the consequences with ever-growing rates of people suffering from premature aging, muscle wasting, diabetes, obesity, and related disorders.

To retain and improve your physical fitness, you must shift back to the low-glycemic foods you were originally programmed for, such as nuts, seeds, legumes, and protein. Minimize the consumption of high-glycemic foods and avoid all sport nutrition and diet products (bars and powders) that are high in sugar or refined carbohydrates.

The glycemic factor is a major determinant of muscle conditioning. Nonetheless, in real life there are many other factors that potentially dictate whether you build or waste your muscle. And there are many important issues that we must address.

For example, what causes your muscle to degrade? And what makes it thrive?

That's next.

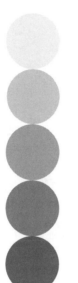

PART II

Muscle Degradation
versus Muscle
Supremacy

Chapter 4

What Causes Your Muscle to Degrade and Age?

Muscle degradation begins in your genes. Scientists identified multiple genes that regulate your physical condition and biological age; most notable among them are those involved in the sustainability of the muscle. It's the decrease in expression of these genes that causes your muscles to deteriorate and age.

Muscle degradation seems to be part of a larger phenomenon. According to the physical laws of thermodynamics, your muscles and body are under constant attack—persistently slammed by the universal forces of entropy. Entropy tries to degrade every living structure on this planet into ash.

To survive that force, you're equipped with a highly sophisticated life-support system that protects your body with an impressive arsenal of life-sustaining compounds. These include your body's own antioxidant peptides and enzymes, immune components, cellular factors, heat-shock proteins, growth factors, and energy molecules—all of which are designed to counteract entropy, rejuvenate tissues, and defeat death.

Life is a constant struggle. Your survival depends on the balance between these opposite forces: rejuvenation versus degradation, life versus death.

As long as the life forces within you are stronger than the forces of degradation, you can keep a youthful appearance and a robust state of health. And every time you heal wounds, restore tissues, or build muscle, you literally beat entropy.

It seems that the power to overcome degradation and death is within you. But how do you take advantage of it? Can you keep your body strong and viable throughout the ages?

Is Aging Inevitable?

Chronological aging starts from the minute you're born. You can't possibly stop the clock from ticking.

But there's also *biological* aging, and growing evidence indicates that this kind of aging can be slowed and even reversed, particularly in the muscle tissue.

The reason is that muscle aging isn't necessarily chronological. A sixty-year-old can have a muscular gene profile similar to that of a person only thirty years old. And a thirty-year-old can already be expressing the genes of a sixty-year-old.

Can Muscle Aging Start at a Young Age?

Muscle aging can start at a young age—as early as the third decade of life. Many young adults may unknowingly be suffering from symptoms of muscle aging, and these become more and more notable as time goes by.

Typically, as a person gets older, the skeletal muscle loses aerobic capacity and strength, as well as size. This is how the vast majority of people today experience aging.

But is it possible to stop that process?

In many respects, it is. But you need to know what triggers the genes that enable your muscle to resist aging.

And note that your daily activities are essential in this process. How you eat, how you exercise, and even how you rest translate into gene activities, and these activities dictate whether you age or stay young.

But to know what to do, you first need to understand what muscle degradation means.

Muscle Degradation

Muscle degradation is a major blow to your body. It's associated with more than just loss of muscle size and strength—muscle degradation can lead to a total metabolic decline.

The biological role of skeletal muscle goes far beyond locomotion. The muscle is responsible for keeping your metabolic system intact. It essentially protects you against obesity, diabetes, and cardiovascular disease. It also enhances your cognitive function and keeps your body young.

Given this, muscle degradation can lead to a major health crisis on a scale far beyond what's commonly thought.

The loss of muscle means a loss of capacity to utilize energy. And a loss of energy means vulnerability to disease, excess weight, and accelerated aging. Muscle degradation seems to be a major factor contributing to the current epidemic of obesity, diabetes, and cardiovascular disease.

It's becoming evidently clear that the benefits you get from your muscular system are essential to your health. Keeping yourself in shape not only makes you feel younger and stronger—it might just save your life.

What Causes Your Muscle to Degrade?

There are many causes of muscle degradation. These include muscle misuse, insulin resistance, hormonal disorders, nutritional deficiencies, inflammatory disease, and aging. But while each of these factors plays a role in muscle degradation, there is growing evidence that they all relate to one underlying cause: *oxidative damage by free radicals.*

Free radicals, known as reactive oxygen species (ROS), are toxic by-products of metabolism. They also invade your body in the form of chemical toxins or rancid food substances. Free radicals lack subatomic particles and are consequently highly reactive as they seek to bind and destroy your cells and tissues.

To defend against these destructive particles, your body uses its endogenous antioxidants along with dietary antioxidants. But when the cumulative concentrations of free radicals overwhelm your body's defenses, oxidative damage to cells and tissues starts taking its toll, destroying cellular proteins, lipids, and nucleic cells.

The accumulated oxidative damage leads to three detrimental changes in the muscle:

- Loss of mitochondrial function
- Loss of neural wiring
- Loss of muscle fibers

The most notable damage occurs in the mitochondria, which is your muscle's energy facility. What are the consequences of mitochondrial damage on your muscle and body? That's next.

Chapter 5

Loss of Mitochondrial Function

The mitochondrion is the energy combustion chamber of the cell. It's an independent cellular organelle that has its own membrane, enzymes, protein, and DNA. Mitochondria are responsible for the utilization of energy for all life functions.

The primary risk to the mitochondria is in the process upon which they utilize energy. Energy utilization in the mitochondria is a brutal event. It involves a molecular exchange of electrons and protons through the mitochondrial inner membrane, and it puts massive oxidative stress on the mitochondria themselves.

To deal with this, your muscle mitochondria are equipped with their own antioxidant enzymes and peptides. But these aren't always sufficient. When oxidative stress surpasses the mitochondria's antioxidant capacity, oxidative damage starts taking its toll, shattering the mitochondrial machinery.

What Causes Accumulated Oxidative Stress?

Oxidative stress can accumulate due to a number of factors, including muscle disuse, aging, chronic overtraining, chronic infection, radiation, chemical toxins, synthetic food additives, nutritional deficiencies, and rancid fat and excessive sugar or fructose intake.

When some of these factors are combined together, the consequences can be detrimental.

For instance, when nutritional deficiencies occur along with chemical toxicity and chronic overtraining, their combined effects could be overwhelmingly destructive, leading to mitochondrial damage in the muscle and a total energy crisis in the body.

The Consequences of Mitochondrial Damage

Mitochondrial damage involves a pathological increase in lipid peroxidation, which destroys the mitochondrial membrane along with cellular proteins and DNA. This is one of the most debilitating side effects of aging.

Consequences of mitochondrial impairment are wide-ranging:

- Impaired capacity to utilize fat and carbohydrates for energy
- Insulin resistance
- Lower threshold for physical exercise
- Excessive weight gain
- Vulnerability to disease

But it doesn't have to be that way. As we'll see later on, there's a way to save your mitochondrial energy system and keep it running strong.

Next we'll take a look at another detrimental aspect of muscle degradation—the loss of neural wiring.

Chapter 6

Loss of Neural Wiring

Your body has a magnificent network of neurons attached to your muscle fibers. Called the neuromuscular system, it controls all your physical actions. But when exposed to accumulated oxidative stress such as due to chronic overtraining, inflammatory disease, or aging, your neural wiring tends to deteriorate.

Consequently, your muscle is rendered weak and dysfunctional like an engine without ignition.

Neuromuscular deterioration is one of the most notable symptoms of aging. It involves gradual disintegration of the junctions between nerve and muscle, and it leads to the loss of motor units along with loss of muscle fibers.

Loss of Motor Units

A motor unit (neuro-motor) is the most basic element of the neuromuscular system. It's a single neural fix, responsible for activating one or many muscle fibers. The more intense and prolonged your physical task is, the more motor units you require. And the more motor units you lose, the weaker and less responsive your muscle becomes.

But it's the fast neuro-motors that you need most. The fast neuro-motors allow you perform intense physical tasks . . . and unfortunately these are first victims of neuromuscular degradation. The fast neuro-motors are most prone to age-related oxidative damage, and their deterioration leads to loss of fast muscle fibers.

Loss of Fast Muscle Fibers

Among your muscle fibers, the fast fibers are the most sensitive to damage. The reason for that is in the way they are wired to their neuro-motors.

Fast muscle fibers are attached to thick cable-like neurons, suitable for intense stimulations and strong contractions. But this highly geared neural-wiring infrastructure is particularly prone to damage by oxidative stress and aging. And its destruction leads to the loss of the fast muscle fiber itself, which again represents a major blow to your physical state.

So what can you do to prevent that loss?

You need to challenge your neuromuscular system. And you need to do this properly.

Challenging Your Neuromuscular System

Your neuromuscular system is programmed to thrive when challenged. It's a highly adaptive system that can either develop or degrade itself depending on how challenged it actually is.

Let me explain.

Each physical task you undertake requires a distinct kind of neural wiring. Take weight lifting, jogging, and walking, for instance. Each of these activities requires a different kind of neural fix. The neurons that stimulate running aren't the same as the neurons that stimulate walking. Similarly, resistance training demands a different neural fix than does aerobics training.

To improve itself, your neuromuscular system must be fully activated. This means that you need to challenge it with multiple tasks. You need to activate as many types of neuro-motors as you can, and particularly your fast neural motors.

The way to do that is first to train intensely and second to incorporate all performance capabilities.

Try to challenge your body intensely with exercises that incorporate strength, speed, and explosive drills. And then try repeating these drills (once or a few times) with minimum rest in between.

The endurance component, as you can see, is inherent to this training regimen.

Note that incorporating strength and speed together is not a common practice. Most exercise programs today lack the complexity and intensity needed for adequately challenging your neuromuscular system.

To sustain and improve your neuromuscular system, you may need to change the way you train. We'll cover this in more detail later on.

Next, let's see why and how you lose muscle fibers.

Chapter 7

Loss of Muscle Fibers

Muscle degradation involves loss of muscle fibers. But it's the deterioration of fast muscle fibers that is most detrimental. That's the main reason why you tend to lose strength and speed as you get older.

So what's the cause of that degradation? And why do you tend to lose fast muscle fibers as you get older?

The loss of fast muscle fibers occurs mainly due to two reasons: inadequate physical challenge and accumulated oxidative damage. Fast muscle fibers are the first to be victimized by the aging process, and they tend to deteriorate due to lack of intense exercise.

But is the loss of fast muscle fibers necessary?

To answer this, we need to take a look at another factor: your muscle genes.

The Genes That Build or Degrade Your Muscle

The fate of your muscle is dictated by genes called myosin heavy chains (MHC genes). These genes are highly sensitive to physical triggers. Any change in your physical conditioning, such as an increase or a decrease in applied strength, is translated into gene activity that can build or waste your muscle fibers.

Simply put, both muscle development and muscle degradation are programmed in your genes. And both depend on your actions or lack of actions.

The MHC genes dictate your physical shape. When triggered, they program and reprogram the neural fix of your muscle fibers. In doing so, they determine how strong or resilient your muscle can be.

But this isn't all.

Incredibly, the MHC genes can also change the character of your muscle fibers. They can literally convert one fiber type to another.

That's a major evolutionary advantage.

The capacity to convert muscle fibers enabled early humans to adapt to extreme physical hardship, which included intense fighting, fleeing, or hunting for hours at a time. This trait allows you today to transform your physique and gain strength and durability without even increasing your muscle size.

But most importantly, the ability to upgrade your muscle fiber quality offers you the means to resist physical aging. With the right physical and nutritional triggers, you can literally improve the quality of your muscle fibers. And yes, you can retain your fast muscle fibers even at an older age.

To understand how this works, we need to take into account another factor: your muscle fiber hierarchy.

What makes one type of muscle fiber biologically superior or inferior to another? And how does this hierarchy affect your muscle fibers' tendency to develop or degrade?

Your Muscle Fiber Hierarchy

Muscle fiber hierarchy is dictated by one key factor: the fiber's quality. To evaluate a muscle fiber's quality, we need to consider two factors: function and fueling capacity.

That raises the question: Which is superior, the fast fibers or the slow fibers?

In terms of function, the fast muscle fibers are stronger and faster than the slow muscle fibers. On the other hand, the slow fibers are more resilient to fatigue.

The slow fibers have a greater capacity to utilize oxygen and sustain aerobic activity because of their larger mitochondrial density and higher blood circulation. In theory, it seems that the slow muscle fibers possess some superior qualities.

But in real life, the slow muscle fibers are simply too slow and too weak.

They don't provide you with the power you need for essential daily activities that require strength or speed. And in times of necessity or danger, which require swift and strong reactions, the slow fibers aren't good enough.

It's the loss of fast muscle fibers that is most devastating to your body. The destruction of fast muscle fibers prohibits you from retaining your muscle size and strength. And as you get older, the fast muscle fibers become even more essential to your vitality.

But note that there are two types of fast muscle fibers. One is superior to the other. And as you'll see soon, the body acknowledges this fiber supremacy, so it tends to preserve it rather than degrade it.

So which muscle fiber is on the top of the hierarchy?

To figure this out we need to take a look at another variable: muscle fueling.

What is muscle fueling? And how does it affect the quality of your muscle fibers? That's next.

Chapter 8

Muscle Fueling

Muscle fueling is one of the most misunderstood factors in sport nutrition. Most people today don't even know what it means.

To keep your muscle strong and viable, you must feed it with the right fuel. If you fail to do that, you'll compromise your muscle's capacity to generate force.

But first, you need to be aware that different muscle fibers require different fuels. As a general rule, the slow muscle fibers have a higher affinity to fat fuel, whereas the fast muscle fibers have different affinities. One is geared almost exclusively to carbohydrate fuel, and the other can utilize both carb and fat fuels.

What dictates the need for a specific fuel is the fiber's enzyme content. Slow muscle fibers have a higher content of fat-metabolizing enzymes, whereas fast muscle fibers have a higher content of carb-metabolizing enzymes.

The following chart presents the fueling capacities and performance capabilities of the different muscle fiber types.

Fueling Capacities of Muscle Fibers

- *Type IIB fast fiber:* Called *fast glycolytic,* this fiber is mostly carb-dependent. The Type IIB fiber is the strongest and fastest, but it lacks durability.
- *Type IIA fast fiber:* Called *fast glycolytic/lipolytic,* this fiber is capable of utilizing both carb and fat fuels. The Type IIA fiber is strong, fast, and durable.

- *Type I slow fiber:* This fiber is classified as *slow lipolytic,* and it predominantly prefers fat fuel. The slow fiber is highly durable but lacks strength and speed.

How Muscle Fueling Affects Your Health

Muscle fueling plays an important role in sustaining your health. Individuals with a high percentage of Type IIB fast muscle fibers have a very limited capacity to utilize fat fuel. This limitation increases their risk for obesity, diabetes, and cardiovascular disorders.

In comparison, people with a high percentage of the Type IIA fast fibers and the Type I slow fibers are less likely to suffer from these health problems, as these fibers are highly efficient at utilizing fat fuel.

Muscle Fueling and Your Fitness Potential

Evidence indicates that there are more than just two types of muscle fibers. Humans are presumably programmed with ten MHC muscle-typing genes, out of which only seven are expressed. This raises an intriguing question: Are we living below our real genetic potential?

And if we do have a higher genetic potential, how can we "wake it up"? Is there a way to literally convert our muscle fibers from normal to superior? Could we possibly transform ourselves from aged and fragile to youthful and robust?

The answer is in your body.

The human body bears proof that we're programmed for a certain degree of physical supremacy. And this potential for supremacy has to do with your muscle's fueling capacity.

Biologically, it seems that we're capable of developing an advanced muscle fiber—a hybrid with superior fueling capacities and unmatched qualities.

What exactly is that hybrid fiber? And can we really develop it? That's next.

Chapter 9

The Super Muscle Fiber

Have you ever wondered what made the ancient Roman and Spartan warriors so incredibly tough?

How could the average 140-pound Roman soldier (fully armed with a sixty-pound gear) endure a daily march of fifteen to thirty miles in rough terrain and then engage in ferocious hand-to-hand combat drills?

And how did the average Spartan warrior endure swinging and slamming a twenty-pound hoplite shield while mastering sword slashing and stabbing for hours at a time? (Try to swing and slam a twenty-pound weight on a punching bag for only three minutes and see how it feels.)

One possible explanation is that these soldiers developed a different muscle fiber than normal people do. Perhaps a super muscle fiber.

So what is that fiber? And does it even exist?

What Is the Super Muscle Fiber?

If there is a super muscle fiber, it isn't yet classified as a type by itself; nor is it officially recognized as a muscle fiber per se. But as you'll soon see, there is a high probability that this fiber indeed exists, most likely as an upgrade hybrid of an already advanced fast muscle fiber, the Type IIA.

What's special about the Type IIA fiber is its unmatched fueling potential. It yields that fiber unmatched capabilities to generate force and resist fatigue.

Let's see how the Type IIA fiber's fueling contributes to its potential supremacy.

Highest Muscle Fiber Quality

Fast muscle fibers are inherently much more energetic than slow fibers. Their energy utilization rates are two to three times greater than those in slow muscle fibers. But as you know, there are two types of fast muscle fibers, and they aren't created equal.

Of the two types, one is apparently more advanced than the other. The Type IIA is better equipped for enduring hardship.

Though the Type IIB fiber is the strongest, biggest, and fastest, it has a profound weakness: low fueling capacity and low durability. Its fueling is limited to mostly carbs, and it can barely utilize fat.

The Type IIA fiber, on the other hand, can utilize both carbohydrate and fat fuels. It has an unmatched capacity to sustain strength, which essentially gives this fast muscle fiber a clear biological advantage.

Most Evolutionarily Advanced Muscle Fiber

Biologist Ki Andersson says in his article "Aspects of Locomotor Evolution in the Carnivore (Mammalia)," that the musculoskeletal system of all mammalian predator species evolved to support their specific hunting behavior.

Humans have been primarily classified as pack hunters. In addition to that, based on shoulder/elbow morphology, humans exhibit features of ambush predators.

This means that beneath our civilized appearance, we're inherently built with distinct predatory features.

As pack hunters, our legs (hind limbs) are designed for long pursuit. And as ambush hunters, our shoulders, elbows, and arms (forelimbs) are built with sufficient range of mobility for grappling and striking.

There seems to be a wolf and a wildcat in each of us. Like wolves, we form packs when engaged in pursuit of a prey or an enemy, and like wildcats we grapple and strike when forced to engage in hand-to-hand fighting.

Our predatory nature seems to be the biological factor that dictates the core of our fitness criteria. Based on that, we need to be strong, fast, and durable at the same time.

The Type IIA fast muscle fiber perfectly fits those criteria.

With its fast contractile power and unique capacity to utilize both carb and fat fuels, the Type IIA fiber can be strong and durable at the same time. No other muscle fiber has those qualities.

Special Durability

Early humans needed special durability. They had to survive intense, prolonged fight-or-flight activities that required highly durable fast muscle fibers. That special durability was a necessity millennia ago.

It has been speculated that our ancestors' muscles were different from ours today. Some anthropologists suggest that early humans' muscles were predominantly made up of more biologically advanced muscle fibers, similar to those found in gorillas.

According to Alan Walker, professor of anthropology and biology at Pennsylvania State University, the difference between modern humans' and great apes' muscle is in the number of motor units. Great apes have fewer but larger motor units than humans.

This enables the great apes to recruit more motor units and generate more force per any given task. In other words, great apes' muscles are predominantly made up of fast muscle fibers, whereas human muscles are made up of both slow and fast muscle fibers. And you can see this in real life.

The average chimpanzee is about five times stronger than a fit, young football athlete. And the average gorilla is estimated to be about ten times stronger than a fit, young human athlete. That's pound for pound.

So does this mean that we're inherently weak?

Not really.

There are known cases of people demonstrating superhuman strength. This phenomenon is called *hysterical strength*.

Hysterical Strength

Hysterical strength is a known phenomenon in which humans exhibit considerably more muscle power than normal. It occurs in cases of people suffering from seizures. And based on anecdotal evidence, it can also occur when people are caught in very stressful survival situations.

There are reports of people being able to do things that would normally be considered impossible, like mothers lifting cars off trapped babies. Or in cases of severe electrical shock, when people are thrown violently by their own extreme muscle contraction.

Why don't we normally express hysterical strength?

One possible explanation has to do with an inherent muscle-inhibitory mechanism in our brain. This cerebral inhibition prevents us from damaging our own bodies with our own muscles. It primarily targets our fast neuro-motors and prohibits our fast muscle fibers from reaching maximum contractile power.

But note that this inhibition is not manifested to the same degree in great apes.

And that tells us something: while great apes still maintain their primordial muscle power, we do not.

According to some biologists, humans have been gradually adapting over the past thousands of years to a weaker muscular system. Our skeleton today is not built to handle the extreme physical hardship that our early ancestors faced. Our ancestors' bodies were more geared for physical power than our bodies are today.

It's plausible, then, that early humans did not have the same muscle-inhibitory mechanism as we do today. Fossil examinations indicate that pound for pound, early humans and Neanderthals were much stronger than we are. Their bodies were highly resilient to stressors that would most likely kill modern humans. But what kind of muscle fibers did these early humans have?

Would these be largely the hybrid Type IIA?

The Type IIA muscle fiber is by far the most biologically advanced. It seems that evolution has led toward the development of this fast muscle fiber in preference to the other fiber types. It's very likely, then, that our ancestors' skeletal muscles were made with high concentrations of that fiber's hybrid.

And the evidence for that seems to exist in your body today.

Most Resilient Muscle Fiber

It's remarkable how your body operates. When intensely and repetitively challenged to physically adapt and improve, your body will convert its fast muscle fibers from one type to another. And it will do that in a very peculiar way.

It transforms muscle fibers in *one* direction only: toward Type IIA.

And not the other way around. It's a one-way street.

Type IIA fibers cannot convert to any other muscle fiber type (except for when you experience an injury or disease). Your body prefers to develop this muscle fiber rather than to degrade it. But could the Type IIA develop into a super muscle fiber? And if so, how?

What Develops Your Type IIA Muscle Fiber?

The main trigger for your Type IIA fiber is extreme repetitive physical challenge. Only extreme physical challenge can affect your muscle-inhibitory mechanism and "wake up" your fast muscle fibers. That's including your Type IIA fiber.

But note again that your body tends to spare your fast muscle fibers from action. It recruits them only when there is no other choice, and it always prefers to use your slow fibers first. That probably serves another purpose: energy conservation. The slow muscle fibers require less energy than the fast fibers. And unless challenged, your body will always tend to conserve its energy.

The point is: you need to counteract that inhibition.

You need to shift your body away from its energy-conserving, muscle-inhibiting mode into a ready-for-action mode. You need to "release the beast"!

How do you do that?

Maximize your challenge by incorporating intense strength and explosive drills and force your body to repeat these drills until you reach a point of virtual paralysis.

When repetitively challenged that way, your Type IIA fiber will be forced to develop into an even stronger, more durable fast muscle fiber. And again, your body will always prefer to build that fiber rather than destroy it. The more trained that fiber gets, the less likely it is that your body will waste it.

Hypothetically, if your muscle is predominantly made up of that advanced fiber, your body will be highly resistant to degradation and aging, and you'll achieve a certain degree of "ancestral" supremacy. That's, of course, in theory.

Is the Super Muscle Fiber Real?

The topic of the hybrid muscle fiber is still in a speculative stage, and it needs to be investigated further. Nonetheless, there is accumulating evidence that the human body possesses more muscle fiber types than was previously thought. On paper, researchers classify these additional muscle fibers as subtypes. But in real life a subtype might very well mean a hybrid.

Given the anecdotes of people exhibiting hysterical strength, there is a high likelihood that the human body is inherently capable of developing an upgraded fast muscle fiber with supreme capabilities. Science is still lagging, though, and there is no conclusive theory that explains the mechanism behind superhuman power. Nonetheless, the hybrid Type IIA muscle fiber is the best clue as to how this phenomenon actually occurs.

Physical supremacy is not an easy goal. It requires determination and a high degree of obsession. Pain is a major factor. And so is time.

What should your muscle protocol be in practice? That's next.

PART III

Your Muscle Protocol

How To Restore and
Rejuvenate Your Muscle

Chapter 10

Your Muscle Protocol

An Overview
Your muscle protocol is based on the following guidelines.

1. Exercise intensely in short intervals.
Short, intense exercise intervals provide your muscle with the right trigger to adapt, improve, and gain size, strength, and durability. And your muscle will respond.

2. For muscle buildup, incorporate small, fast-assimilating, low-glycemic protein meals throughout the day.
Incorporating small, fast-assimilating, low-glycemic protein meals throughout the day allows the highest protein utilization in your muscle with minimum side effects on your insulin and digestive system.

3. For muscle rejuvenation, exercise while fasting and have your recovery meal after exercise.
Exercise while fasting activates genes and growth factors that recycle your muscle tissues. Feeding your muscle after exercise will stop muscle catabolism and shift the recycling process toward recovery and growth.

4. Increase your antioxidant intake from food.
Increased intake of antioxidant food nutrients provides your muscle with the extra protection it needs against oxidative damage.

5. Maintain a low-glycemic and satiety-oriented diet.
Base your diet on satiety foods to support your body's metabolism and keep your hormonal and muscular systems intact.

Note that the above guidelines must be followed properly. If you overlook even one of them, your progress will be compromised. To get results, the physical element must be combined with the nutritional elements.

Next we'll overview your training protocol.

Chapter 11

The Short Intense Training Protocol

Each of us engages in short, intense physical activities. We do that when we climb stairs, move heavy objects, unscrew a stubborn jar lid, or strike a punch. Short, intense activities are essential to our species' fight-or-flight apparatus. Without this physical capacity we can't independently survive. So we must keep it intact.

What Is the Short Intense Training Protocol? And How Can It Help You?

The Short intense training protocol aims at developing strength and special durability at the same time. It targets your fast neuro-motors with short, intense, repetitive challenges while minimizing the risk of oxidative damage in your muscle.

Compared to other fitness approaches, this training protocol offers you by far the greatest benefits. These include:

- Restoring your muscle's work output
- Sparing your muscle from wasting
- Sparing your mitochondria from damage
- Keeping your fast neuro-motors intact
- Increasing your muscle mass
- Increasing your muscle's glycogen-loading capacity
- Improving your body composition

Let's see how these benefits are manifested in real life and take a look at what makes this training protocol superior to others.

Restoring Your Muscle's Work Output

Typically, your muscle's work output decreases with age, but that capacity can be restored and even increased by short intense training.

Studies have shown that short intense training increases muscle work output at any age, but remarkably, it has been shown to have an even greater beneficial effect on older people (12.5-percent power gain in sixty- to seventy-year-olds versus 8-percent power gain in twenty- to thirty-year-olds).

These findings prove how responsive aged muscle is to short intense training.

Triggering a Mechanism That Spares Your Muscle from Wasting

Incredibly, your muscle has a self-preservation mechanism. This mechanism, which actually protects your active muscle from breaking down, can be triggered by short intense training.

Short, repetitive bouts of intense weight lifting have been shown to help counteract age-related muscle waste. Note that this effect is substantially less notable in moderate training.

Exercise intensity is essential to sparing your muscle from wasting. It's the intensity element that keeps your fast muscle fibers intact.

Scientists believe that the signal to retain the muscle has to do with acute depletion of muscle energy, which is typically associated with short, intense exercise intervals.

But to get results, both elements of the exercise protocol must be applied. Both the *short* and the *intense* have to be incorporated properly. "Short" means short in duration (seconds to minutes). "Intense" means maximal or submaximal levels of exercise intensity.

Increasing Your Muscle's Glycogen-Loading Capacity

The short intense training protocol can help increase your muscle's capacity for glycogen loading. And in this respect, it can benefit men and women alike.

In just twelve weeks, this exercise protocol has been shown to produce a significant 27-percent increase in women's muscle glycogen. It also helped restore age-related oxygenation decline, improve fiber quality, and increase muscle mass.

Truly, this is the only training approach that could potentially benefit all sport conditioning programs.

Let's continue and see how this protocol can help you counteract the main determinants of muscle degradation.

Sparing Your Muscle Mitochondria from Damage

The loss of mitochondrial function in your muscle is caused by accumulated oxidative damage. That's the main reason why your exercise threshold typically decreases as you age. By limiting the duration of the workout, there's less chance for accumulation of excessive free radicals in the mitochondria. Hence, a lower risk for mitochondrial damage.

In comparison, chronic prolonged low-intensity exercise sessions tend to overwhelm your mitochondrial defenses. This type of training puts your mitochondria and muscle at a high risk of damage.

And this risk seems to increase as you get older.

Chronic prolonged exercise sessions can be especially countereffective to people who have just started or resumed training. Gym classes and personal training routines that run for prolonged durations (i.e., one hour or more) are often beyond the exercise threshold of the trainees.

Keeping Your Fast Neuro-Motors Intact

Short, intense exercise intervals can help counteract neuro-motor degradation. Studies in older women who undertook twelve weeks of short, intense resistance-training intervals showed a 20-percent increase in muscle cross-sectional area.

This remarkable gain occurred largely due to fast muscle fiber's hypertrophy, which is a clear indication of fast neuro-motor preservation.

Improving Your Muscle Fiber Quality

Recent research indicated that the short intense training protocol can help improve muscle fiber quality. And again this improvement is not limited to age or gender. When the short intense training protocol is undertaken, the percentage of Type IIB fibers decreases as the percentage of Type IIA fibers increases, which indicates an improvement in fast muscle fiber composition.

But incredibly, the Type IIB fast muscle fibers aren't the only ones that upgrade their quality. Researchers have found that even the Type I slow muscle fibers become faster in response to short, intense physical challenges. And this increase in contractile speed occurred because of the improved fiber's neural wiring.

The result is that your supposedly "slow" muscle fibers can now develop in a way that will allow them to mimic fast fibers. That again indicates a substantial improvement in muscle fiber quality and performance.

Could this be the right protocol to achieve muscle supremacy?

We'll continue addressing this in your workout. That's next.

Chapter 12

Your Workout

Your workout regimen is based on repetitive drills that combine strength, speed, and explosive elements. The endurance element is inherent to this regimen.

Why Do You Need to Combine Strength, Speed, and Endurance?

The combined impact of strength, speed, and endurance works a larger variety of fast neuro-motors than does conventional strength or endurance training. This approach goes against the typical trend. Most people don't combine strength and speed together, and endurance training is generally done in a separate session. Nonetheless, that's what is essentially needed to trigger your Type IIA fast muscle fiber to develop and improve.

Let's look a little closer at these terms:

- **Strength:** the capacity to resist an applied force
- **Speed:** the capacity to incorporate fast repetitive moves
- **Endurance:** the capacity to resist fatigue

The combined effect of strength, speed, and endurance is essential to your fitness regardless to your age. Strength and speed training increases your muscle's force production, whereas endurance training increases your muscle's oxidative capacity.

And it gets even better when you add explosive elements.

That's the ultimate challenge.

Under such a challenge, your body will be forced to upgrade your fast muscle fibers in favor of the more advanced Type IIA fiber. Remember, that's the only fiber that can handle strength, speed, and endurance drills combined.

Finally, this type of training fully accommodates your core fitness criteria (see Chapter 9). It's the only way to get you stronger, faster, and more durable altogether.

Your Exercise Drills

The combined effect of strength, speed, and explosive elements is highly demanding, especially when you need to repetitively endure that in several interval drills.

Following are examples of such drills:

 I. Combine heavy weight lifting with speed punching.
 II. Combine heavy weight lifting with explosive, light weight lifting.
 III. Combine squat exercise with a jump-rope drill.
 IV. Combine squat exercise with jump kicks (jump kicks can be done in front of a punching bag or just in the air).
 V. Combine squat exercise with sprinting (such as fast running in place).

To work your upper and lower body, combine drill I with drill IV or combine drill II with drill V.

Try these additional options:

• Add pull-ups to each of your drills.
• Do your squat exercise while holding a barbell or dumbbells overhead in a straight-hand position.

Make your intervals short, around one to three minutes. And then repeat them with minimum rest in between—fifteen to thirty seconds. Your workout should not exceed thirty minutes. If you feel you can go beyond that, you probably haven't trained intensely enough.

What Should You Expect in Return?

Expect improvements in your strength, speed, explosive capacities, and durability. Within a few weeks you'll notice how your body gets harder and leaner. Yes, that's if you're ready to continue taking this routine on yourself.

But note that strength seems to contradict speed. So when combining the two, your maximum performance may initially be affected. However, when resuming sheer strength or speed training, you may actually notice improvements in both performance capabilities over your starting point. And that's with the bonus of increased durability.

Let me be clear:

Ten minutes of this training regimen can yield better results than an hour of a low-intensity workout. In fact, even three minutes of this regimen will be perceived by your body as a stronger signal to adapt and improve (see below).

Your Workout Guidelines

1. **Work your whole body.** Exercise as many muscle groups as possible. Compound exercises are always superior to isolated exercises. And the benefits you get from free weight training are unmatched to those you get from exercise machines.

2. **Keep your workout short.** The short intense training protocol allows you to fully challenge your body within three to thirty minutes. There is no need to go beyond that.

3. **Try the three-minute "killer" workout.** You can blast a full workout in only three minutes. Yes, three minutes of this special regimen will get you better results than sixty minutes of a low-intensity workout. That's if you're ready to endure extreme hardship nonstop for three minutes.

- *The Three-Minute Stairs Drill.* This drill requires you to go up and down the stairs nonstop for three minutes while lifting weights.

You can do this facing forward, or you can try going up and down the stairs backward. In any case, adjust the rhythm of your legs to your hands (e.g., "left leg–right hand," etc.). And be careful when you go up and down the stairs backward. Make sure you step properly and keep your balance. Also, choose weights that you can handle for the full length of the drill.

- *The Three-Minute Running with Weights Drill.* This is another short, killer workout. Pick up lightweight dumbbells and step on a treadmill. Hold the weights above your head in a straight hand position and run for a thirty-second interval. Follow that with another thirty-second interval in which you hold the weights in front of your forehead (similar to a boxer's defense position). Repeat these intervals until you complete a three-minute drill. Adjust the weight load and speed level to accommodate your physical capacity. If you feel that running with weights is too intense, try walking with weights instead, but keep your hands in the two positions described above.

4. **Intensity is a relative term.** Each of us has a physical threshold. For one person, max intensity means lifting two hundred pounds, while for another person it might be only twenty pounds. Here is how you can figure out your maximum intensity level.

For resistance training, choose a weight you can lift no more than five times. Or in turn, choose light weights that you can barely endure in a nonstop three-minute drill.

And you can also train intensely without weights. For instance, you can do explosive exercises such as power or speed punching, or push and pull drills, but whatever you're doing, go all way out.

And how do you know whether you reached your maximum intensity threshold? Simply, your pain will tell you. That's until you get nauseated or reach a point of virtual paralysis.

5. **Try a variety of speed exercise.** For instance, you can try running in one place, or running up and down the stairs. Or perhaps try sprinting

outdoors. For your upper body, use explosive punching drills, or swipe a towel up and down similar to dusting a rug, or do both. Then check how you score in each drill. Count how fast your feet hit the ground per fixed time, or how fast you run up and down the stairs, or how fast you can sprint outdoors. Similarly, check how fast you punch per fixed time or how many times you can swipe a towel per fixed time. Write down your scores and use them as a reference to monitor your progress.

6. **Increase the level of your challenge.** As you get stronger, you'll notice how your training feels easier and easier. This indicates that you need to upgrade your physical challenge. You can do that by increasing your weight load or speed level or by increasing the duration of your drill. Also, try to increase your level of difficulty. For instance, try lifting and punching while standing on one leg. Alternatively, you can incorporate the same drill but do your punching with weights. You'll feel the difference.

7. **Don't take on more than you can handle.** If you increase your weight load or speed, don't try to increase your exercise duration at the same time. If you increase your exercise duration (longer drills or more intervals), don't increase your weight load or speed. Only when you notice substantial progress in all your performance capabilities should you try increasing the weight load, speed, and duration at the same time.

8. **Wake up your fast neuro-motors to jump start your day.** A short, intense morning drill of only two to three minutes can do the job. You can do intense weight lifting, towel swiping, power/speed punching, or sprinting. This will shift your body away from an energy-conserving, inhibitory mode into a ready-for-action mode.

9. **Change the order of your exercise.** For instance, if you like starting your workout with strength drills followed by explosive drills, change the order of your exercise to start with explosive drills followed by strength drills. This change will challenge your muscles to further adapt and improve.

10. **Don't train seven days a week.** Take a break once or twice per week. This will allow your body to fully recuperate. Remember, exercise is for challenge, and rest is for recovery. And you need both to succeed.

Remember, your exercise regimen is only part of your muscle protocol. I know people who exercise intensely every other day, but they don't look fit or healthy. And the reason: inadequate nutrition.

To effectively transform your physique, you need to know how to feed your muscle.

Your nutritional protocol is next.

Chapter 13

Your Nutritional Protocol

The premise of your nutritional protocol is to enable your muscle to build up and keep it from wasting.

Your muscle can waste due to two kinds of nutritional deficiencies:

1. Protein
2. Antioxidant

When your muscle-protein uptake is too low, your muscle breaks more protein than it deposits, and it consequently loses size and strength. When your antioxidant uptake is insufficient, your muscle's defenses may get overwhelmed by oxidative free radicals, which may start destroying and wasting your tissues.

To protect your muscle from wasting and oxidative damage, you need to feed it with sufficient protein and antioxidants from whole, fresh, and chemical-free food sources.

But to practically choose the right foods for your muscle, you need to first know what muscle nourishment means.

Muscle Nourishment

Muscle nourishment is not a typical feeding. It isn't about shoving in protein, fat, or carbs and then expecting results—this is a skill that requires knowledge and practice.

Everything about the way you eat is important. Every single factor— from your choice of food and the timing of your meals to the way you combine your foods—can affect how your muscle assimilates nutrients, utilizes energy, and develops.

Each of these factors contributes to your physical state.

The art of muscle nourishment has largely been lost to us. Despite the ever-growing number of people taking up fitness and sports activities, our society is still not "muscle oriented."

But perhaps this is quite understandable. After all, we're not as dependent on muscle power as our ancestors were centuries and millennia ago. And there's also the fact that proper muscle nourishment requires a certain level of sophistication, which is beyond mainstream knowledge.

As technologically oriented as you may be, you need to be aware that your fitness is not. To figure out what benefits your muscle, you need to stop looking for future technologies and instead look back to the past.

Our ancestors didn't have the benefits of modern science and technology, yet we now know that they were stronger and more durable than we are today. Which tells you something important: human fitness is inherently primitive. And there's nothing "modern" about it.

There are no quick fixes or gimmicks when it comes to feeding your muscle. There is no super-advanced, engineered food or miracle pill that can do the job for you.

The Five Essential Components of Your Nutritional Protocol

Your nutritional protocol is made up of five essential components.

1. **Your protein source:** finding the right protein for your muscle.
2. **The glycemic impact of your meals:** controlling the glycemic impact of your meals for proper utilization of nutrients and energy.
3. **Your fuel choice:** choosing the right fuel for your muscle's needs.
4. **Your meal size and timing:** making sure you're eating the right food at the right time and at the right amount.
5. **Your antioxidant intake:** increasing your body's antioxidant defenses to ward off muscle degradation.

Next we'll take a close look at each of your nutritional protocol's components, starting with your protein choice.

Chapter 14

Your Protein Choice

Your muscle consumes and spends more protein than any other tissue. It demands at least as much protein as it loses each day. And if your daily protein intake is insufficient, your muscle will start wasting itself.

But insufficient protein intake isn't the only reason why your muscle breaks down. Muscle waste often occurs due to bad protein choices.

If your protein is from an inferior source or if it's damaged by heat or acid processing, it won't fully nourish your muscle. An inferior protein won't provide your muscle with all the amino acids and nutritional cofactors it needs. As a result, your muscle will be forced to dig into its own tissue to retrieve the missing elements.

Your protein quality is critically important. It can make the difference between progress and failure. You can consume enormous amounts of inferior protein and see no results, and with only moderate amounts of quality protein, you can get great results.

What Does Your Muscle Need in a Protein?

Your muscle requires a protein food that is complete and whole. It should contain all the key amino acids along with nutritional cofactors such as naturally occurring vitamins, minerals, immune components, antioxidants, and naturally occurring fuel. Your protein choice should be fresh, minimally processed, chemical-free, and easily digestible.

In its whole-food form, protein is always attached to its naturally occurring cofactors such as minerals, vitamins and fuel components, fat or carbs, or both. And it never comes in the form of "protein isolate."

You can't afford to overlook this. The nutritional cofactors play essential roles in protein utilization and energy production. They support your body's acid/base balance as well as your muscle's antioxidant defenses—they're crucially needed for your body's metabolic integrity.

Being complete, whole, fresh, chemical-free, minimally processed, and digestible—that's your protein criteria.

What Proteins Don't Fit the Criteria?

All protein isolates, including whey isolate, milk isolate, soy isolate, rice isolate, hemp isolate, and virtually all other commercial plant proteins, are overly processed and devoid of nutritional cofactors. Hence, they don't fit the protein criteria.

And there are some protein sources that seem to fit the criteria, but they're nevertheless problematic. So let's see what fits your muscle and what doesn't.

Do Animal-Flesh and Marine Foods Fit Your Muscle Needs?

Technically, all animal-flesh and marine foods including meat, poultry, eggs, dairy, fish, and seafood are complete proteins. And they seem to fit your muscle needs. Plant foods, on the other hand, are considered incomplete and therefore inferior choices.

But that's not always the case. When combined properly, plant proteins can actually match animal proteins in their nutritional viability and muscle-building properties.

In reality, however, only a few protein foods in our typical diet actually fulfill the criteria for muscle nourishment. And contrary to common belief, most proteins from animal-flesh and marine foods aren't really complete.

Let me explain.

You probably like eating your meat or fish cooked, and you may enjoy the taste of it. But what fits your palate doesn't necessarily fit your muscle. The truth is, cooking and processing damage important amino acids and render the protein deficient and inferior.

And there is another concern. Unless labeled as organic, animal-fresh foods are likely polluted with hormones, antibiotics, pesticides, and chemical additives. Similarly, marine foods raise some serious concerns. Unless wild catch from deep or north seas, they're typically polluted with high levels of mercury and dangerous petrochemicals.

For a person who already suffers from a compromised immune system, conventional animal-flesh and marine foods are far from being the ideal choices.

Animal-flesh and marine foods are slow to digest and slow to assimilate, which makes them unsuitable for muscle recovery after exercise.

After exercise, your muscle requires fast-assimilating proteins. Only fast-assimilating proteins can swiftly block the catabolic effect of exercise and shift your muscle into an anabolic state. Slow-digesting proteins can't do that—they can't accommodate your muscle needs after exercise.

But this doesn't mean that you shouldn't eat slow-assimilating animal or marine foods.

It just indicates that these foods are not viable for postexercise recovery. Slow-digesting animal foods can certainly benefit your muscle if you eat them at the right time. And if you choose to eat them, make sure your meat is fresh from organic grass-fed animal sources, and your fish is wild catch, preferably from deep or north seas.

Another option is eating animal foods raw or cured. Eating raw fish or meat may seem scary and risky today, but you can get naturally cured fish or meat. This is a viable way to grant the integrity of the protein and improve its digestibility. Of course, that's if your food source is fresh and carefully handled.

Note that animal-flesh and marine foods provide your body with a powerful muscle-protective compound not found in plant foods. Called carnosine, this compound acts to protect your muscle protein from degradation due to glycation, cross-linking, or racemization. Your body can produce carnosine from nucleotides or from beta alanine, a special protein found in animal and marine foods.

What's the Case with Eggs and Cheese?

On paper, eggs and cheese are great protein foods with impressive nutritional profiles. But in real life they're typically served after being heated. Eggs are generally eaten cooked, and cheese products are typically derived from pasteurized milk. Eggs and cheese are also slow to digest and assimilate. Hence, eggs and cheese are not your best choices for muscle recovery after exercise.

But then again, that doesn't mean you shouldn't eat them. Choose eggs from free-range chickens and organic cheese preferably from raw milk. In fact, even conventional eggs and cheese provide high concentrations of the muscle-building branched-chain amino acids (BCAAs), including leucine.

Again, eggs, cheese, meat, poultry, and marine foods can fully benefit your muscle if you eat them at the right time. We'll cover this in more detail later on. Meanwhile, we're left with one question:

What's the Ideal Protein Choice for Your Muscle?

There is no ideal protein choice for your muscle. Each protein has its pros and cons. Nonetheless, taking into account all the criteria for muscle nourishment, and based on accumulating scientific data, there is one protein source that seems to surpass all others.

Not only can this protein benefit your muscle, but it can also be used at any time, and particularly after exercise. A component of milk called whey protein, it's the fastest to assimilate among all protein foods and the most nourishing.

Let's take a closer look at whey protein and how it benefits your muscle.

Chapter 15

Whey Protein

Whey is a by-product of cheese manufacturing. It was initially discarded as waste or used for animal feed, but later on scientists discovered that it was an outstandingly beneficial food. Not only was whey found to be a most viable protein source, but it has also gained a reputation as one of the most powerful immunosupportive foods available.

The nutritional properties of whey are truly remarkable. But to make use of them, you have to be careful about the whey that you choose. Not all whey products are the same.

Unfortunately, most whey products today are derived from ultrapasteurized milk of factory-farm cows. These products are typically overly processed, overheated, and damaged. Also, beware of products labeled as whey isolate. These are devoid of vital nutritional cofactors and therefore don't fit the criteria of quality protein.

The protein industry is a booming business. To maximize profitability, many manufacturers choose to produce cheap proteins often drenched with chemical additives and toxic substances. Based on 2010 consumer reports, some of the most popular whey protein brands in the United States were found to contain alarming concentrations of heavy metals. That's including cadmium, arsenic, and lead.

Quality is not a concern when money is the main motive. To make you buy their product, protein distributors use false claims supported by pseudoscience. The truth is that most commercial proteins today, including whey products, are unfit for human consumption (or even animal consumption).

Quality whey is a rare commodity these days. To be classified as quality whey, the product has to be whole, cold-processed, and derived from the raw milk of grass-fed cows. There are very few whey products that fit this category.

So what's special about grass-fed cows' whey? What are the specific properties of quality whey? And how do you choose your whey?

What's Special about Grass-Fed Cows' Whey?

It has been widely proven that grass-fed cows' dairy has a superior nutritional value compared to conventional dairy. Pasture-grazing cows are healthier than grain-fed cows. They're commonly raised by small family farms that care about their animals' health. That's in contrast with farm factory cows, which are commonly caged, inhumanely treated, overcrowded, overstressed, grain fed, and injected with antibiotics and hormones.

Grass-fed cows' milk is certainly healthier than grain-fed cows' milk. It's richest in immunosupportive nutrients, antioxidants, and metabolic enhancing proteins. And nowhere is this nutritional supremacy better demonstrated than in grass-fed cows' whey.

Let's take a closer look at the unique properties of quality whey.

Complete Profile of Amino Acids

Pound for pound, the protein profile in whole, unheated whey is more impressive than any other food on the planet. It provides the largest spectrum of essential and conditionally essential amino acids, and it's remarkably high in the muscle-building branched-chain amino acids (BCAAs), particularly leucine. Whey protein is also rich in glutamic acid, which plays an important role in muscle buildup.

Quality whey protein has a similar composition to human breast milk. It's an exclusive source of immunosupportive compounds, antioxidant peptides, and metabolic enhancing nutrients. And like breast milk, it can help support growth and rejuvenation.

Exclusive Source of the Immuno-Peptide Glutamylcysteine

Whole, unheated whey protein is an exclusive source of glutamylcysteine, which is the most bioactive form of cysteine. The amino acid cysteine is missing in most protein foods commonly destroyed by cooking and processing. But your body requires this amino acid; it's essential for all your immuno functions. What's special about glutamylcysteine is its unmatched immune-boosting properties. It acts like a "super cysteine."

Glutamylcysteine is instantly converted by your body to the antioxidant peptide glutathione. That's your body's most important immuno molecule. Glutathione is crucially needed for all major detoxification and immune activities. It has been widely regarded as a marker of health.

High levels of glutathione indicate a prime state of health, whereas low levels of glutathione are linked to immune deficiencies, disease, and aging.

In times of high physical stress, injury, or disease, your body typically loses its cysteine pool along with its ability to produce glutathione. This means that you need to consume more cysteine-rich foods to support your physically active lifestyle. And you need this amino acid particularly as you age, since it helps counteract the aging process.

Let's take a look at how critical cysteine is.

Cysteine and Your Physical Shape

Cysteine is vital for your physical shape. It's also one of the key amino acids used to ward off disease and aging. In its naturally occurring form, cysteine has been shown to

- decrease your body fat percentage while increasing muscle mass;
- increase the cellular level of glutathione peroxidase, which is your body's most powerful antioxidant enzyme;
- increase your muscle endurance;
- decrease risk for oxidative damage in your muscle mitochondria.

Plasma concentrations of cysteine and its metabolite glutathione have been shown to be prognostic of increased lean body mass.

In summary, cysteine is essential to increasing muscle mass, decreasing body fat, and protecting against cellular oxidative damage. That's the Holy Grail of human fitness. And whey's cysteine helps you reach that.

But note that this is not exactly the case with synthetic cysteine.

Unlike whey's cysteine, the synthetic N-acetyl-cysteine is unable to cross the muscle's cell membrane (sarcolemma). And it's therefore unable to increase glutathione levels within the cell.

Furthermore, when taken in large dosages, N-acetyl-cysteine has been shown to have side effects, including gastrointestinal disorders and blurred vision. The naturally occurring cysteine in whey is undoubtedly superior and safer as compared to its synthetic equivalents.

Beware of Cysteine Deficiencies

Deficiencies of cysteine along with other key amino acids such as lysine and carnitine are highly prevalent today. Cysteine and lysine, for instance, are easily damaged by heat and acid processing and therefore are largely missing in our typical diet.

But your body desperately needs these amino acids. They play key roles in keeping your metabolism intact, and they contribute to your muscle's energy production and durability.

Quality whey protein can help prevent these deficiencies. Whole, unheated, grass-fed cows' whey protein is the most viable source of cysteine and other fragile amino acids commonly missing in our diet.

Let's continue with the properties of whey protein.

Immuno Support

Whole, unheated whey protein contains the most impressive spectrum of immunosupportive, antioxidant, and anticancerous compounds of all foods. Again, similar immune compounds are found in human breast milk, where they play essential roles in protecting the newborn against infections and disease.

These include immunoglobulins, alpha-lactoglobulins, bovine serum albumin, lactoferrin, glycomacropeptides, and conjugated linoleic acids (CLAs).

The immune-boosting effects of whey protein have been widely documented to greatly benefit individuals with compromised immunity as well as athletes engaged in intense physical training and people recovering from injury.

Fast Nutrient Delivery

One of whey protein's most important properties is fast nutrient delivery. This trait makes whey protein most suitable for muscle recovery after exercise.

As noted, after exercise, your muscle is at peak capacity to utilize nutrients, and that's when you need to feed it with fast-assimilating proteins. Whey protein can perfectly accommodate this window of opportunity. It yields the fastest anabolic impact on your muscle.

But to fully benefit from all these outstanding health properties, you need to be able to choose your whey. Only quality whey can grant you desirable results.

How to Choose Your Whey

To make sure the whey product you're getting is truly viable, use the following guidelines:

- Your whey should be free of pesticides, chemicals, and GMO ingredients.
- Your whey should be derived from grass-fed, non-hormone-treated cows.
- Your whey should be unheated and non-acid-treated. Both heat and acid processing damage amino acids, rendering the whey insoluble and inferior.
- Beware of whey protein isolates. These products are overly processed, often treated with heat and acid, and they typically

have a funky taste. The human body has never adapted to consume protein in an isolate form. And there are some concerns regarding possible toxic side effects.

- Use only quality whey protein concentrate. It's a whole food, and it contains all the nutritional cofactors, including minerals, lipids, and immune components, which are typically lost in whey isolate. Whey protein concentrate is yet lower in fat and lactose, and it has a richer, creamier taste.
- Beware of whey products with poor solubility. This indicates damaged amino acids and inferior quality. When amino acids are damaged or denatured, they lose their original water-soluble configuration. Insoluble whey is a degraded product with a typical acid aftertaste.
- Avoid whey products containing synthetic additives, artificial sweeteners, sugar alcohol, or fructose. These substances affect your body as toxins, often with harmful side effects.
- Avoid whey products made with hydrolyzed proteins. Hydrolyzation and fermentation of protein yields MSG and damages fragile immune components.

Though a superfood, whey protein is only one component of your diet. In real life, you need to know how to select and combine a variety of protein foods, particularly those that are commonly part of your diet.

How to combine proteins? That's next.

Chapter 16

How to Combine Proteins

Each of us combines proteins just by the simple act of preparing a meal. But to do that in a way that actually benefits your muscle, you need to know how to evaluate proteins and how to match them.

Evaluating Proteins

Protein foods are generally qualified according to their biological value (BV). Biological value is measured by taking into account three variables: the protein's amino acid score, digestibility, and effect on growth.

But there is something peculiar about the biological value of protein blends.

A blend of proteins will always yield the same or greater biological value than each of the blend's components. This means that a protein blend will never yield a lower biological value than that of each of the blend's components.

Scientists speculate that this phenomenon has to do with the fact that humans adapted to better utilize protein from a mixed food diet, which may have played an important evolutionary purpose. During primordial times of famine or low food supply, gathering foods from various scarce sources allowed humans to get the maximum biological value from the minimum protein available.

Matching Proteins

To get the highest biological value, you need to select proteins that complement each other. Complementary proteins enhance each other's nutritional value with their amino acid, fat, vitamin, or mineral content.

Examples of protein sources that complement each other include rice and beans, peas and potatoes, eggs and cheese, fish and lentils, meat and nuts, and beans and seeds.

Each of these blends yields a better amino score and a superior nutritional profile than that of their individual components.

However, just as there are proteins that increase each other's value, there are some that don't.

For instance, a blend of slow-digesting animal-flesh proteins, such as meat and chicken or turkey and pork, yields a value no higher than that of the individual components. Such combinations are generally less digestible and more likely to cause reactions.

So what's the most viable way to combine proteins?

Mix animal proteins with plant proteins.

That combination never fails. Virtually every mixture of animal protein and plant protein increases the nutritional value of the blend. Combinations of meat, fish, or eggs with legumes, roots, nuts, or seeds always yield greater health properties than those of animal proteins or plant proteins alone.

So how do you time your protein blends?

Timing Your Protein Blends

Your body needs different types of proteins throughout the circadian clock. During the day it needs fast-assimilating proteins, whereas at night it needs more slow-assimilating proteins.

Fast-assimilating proteins readily nourish your body during the day with minimum digestive stress, and they're particularly essential for muscle recovery after exercise. During the night, however, there is a greater need for slow-assimilating proteins, which can grant a slow, steady release of amino acids to your muscle and a long-lasting anabolic effect during the sleeping hours.

Protein Blends for Daytime

The foods that fit this category most are fast-assimilating dairy products from cows, goats, or sheep. These include yogurt, kefir, milk, and whey. Whey protein is the fastest to assimilate among them and has the highest biological value.

Sheep and goat milks are known for their excellent protein matrix. They're high in alpha-lactalbumin, a major immune component of human breast milk that is found in smaller amounts in bovine milk.

So how do you combine these fast-assimilating proteins?

Start with whey protein and combine it with the other fast-assimilating protein sources. For instance, a combination of whey with yogurt or milk will yield an excellent protein blend. These combinations not only have the highest biological value but also complement each other with their nutritional cofactors. They yield a richer taste, as well. Such blends are highly effective for recovery after exercise.

(For those who can't tolerate dairy, see "Protein Blends for the Dairy Sensitive" below.)

But there is one blend that could yield an even superior value. It's a combination of two kinds of whey protein: whey protein concentrate and sweet whey.

Whey Protein Concentrate and Sweet Whey

On their own, each of these proteins has a great biological value. But when mixed together, they yield an even superior blend.

The first component is whey protein concentrate. Typically constituted with 80-percent protein, the concentrate provides all the key amino acids along with all whey's immune fragments and nutritional cofactors. Whey protein concentrate should be the largest component in the blend.

The second component is sweet whey, also known as native whey. A minimally processed whole native whey, it's pound for pound the most viable source of minerals and nutritional cofactors needed for protein utilization.

Sweet whey is also a great prebiotic food. It supports healthy gut bacteria, which are essential for protein digestion and utilization, and has been used by Swiss physicians as a digestive aid and health remedy. Sweet whey is a highly mineralized food that cannot be consumed in large quantities. It should therefore be the smaller component in the mixture.

Combining these two whey proteins will yield a blend with the highest biological value and highest digestibility. And it will yield a richer, creamier taste.

Protein Blends for Nighttime

As we've seen, your muscle needs slow-assimilating proteins during the night.

The best slow-assimilating protein blends are made with animal and plant proteins. These blends will always yield a high biological value and a great nutritional profile.

But when needed, you can also combine plant proteins alone or combine animal proteins alone.

The best plant protein blends are

- Legumes and seeds
- Legumes and nuts
- Legumes and grains
- Peas and potatoes

The best animal protein blends are

- Cheese and eggs
- Fish and eggs
- Fish and cheese

Meat and eggs is also a viable combination, but it's less digestible and therefore less desirable.

Note that eggs should be eaten whole with the yolk. Egg yolk has a better amino acid composition than egg white, with 50 percent more leucine to trigger muscle growth.

Protein Blends for the Dairy Sensitive

Some people are sensitive to milk, mostly due to lactose intolerance. Surprisingly, though, a large percentage of dairy-sensitive people can tolerate moderate servings of whey protein. That's because whey protein is generally low in lactose.

If, however, you're dairy intolerant, your best alternatives to whey protein are poached or lightly cooked eggs and raw fish (sashimi) as naturally cured. But note that these aren't as fast assimilating as liquid dairy proteins. And they can only combine with themselves or with plant proteins, which are also slow assimilating.

Other alternatives are combinations of marine food, meat, or poultry with vegetarian protein foods. But again, all these are slow assimilating and therefore won't be ideal for postexercise recovery.

Protein Blends for Vegans

If you're a vegan, your best options are proper combinations of plant foods such as legumes and seeds (humus), legumes and nuts, peas and potatoes, and beans and grains. Note that sprouted beans and grains yield a higher nutritional value and faster nutrient delivery than their conventional equivalents.

However, legumes, seeds, nuts, and grains are slow to digest and slow to assimilate. And even though these are whole and healthy, they aren't as efficient as whey protein for muscle nourishment during the day, and they're certainly not as effective in promoting muscle recovery after exercise.

Avoid Dairy Imitations

Stay clear of all dairy imitations. Especially beware of products made with soy protein. Soy protein has been shown to cause metabolic disorders in sensitive individuals due to its inherent estrogenic activity. Supermarket shelves are packed with fake dairy and meat products. These include imitations of milk, cheese, and meat made with soy or rice protein isolates. These fake foods are always overly processed, and their nutritional value is worthless.

For muscle and body nourishment, always eat a real food rather than a fake one.

Combining protein is important, but there is another critical factor to which you need to pay attention. That's the glycemic loads of your meal.

If you overlook that, you may jeopardize the viability of your diet.

Chapter 17

The Glycemic Load
of Your Meal

Glycemic load is a term that describes the effect of food on blood sugar. The higher the glycemic load, the more it spikes your blood sugar and insulin. There has been a growing public awareness to the glycemic factor and how it affects our health. Nevertheless, this has been one of the most misunderstood issues, particularly in the area of sport nutrition.

One of the most common fallacies is that high-glycemic protein meals promote muscle gain. Commercial protein products are often packed with a high sugar content, claiming to deliberately spike insulin and thereby promote muscle gain. It has been speculated that since insulin is an anabolic hormone, it will promote protein deposit in the muscle when overspiked. That's the idea . . . but that's not what happens in real life.

In real life, high-glycemic protein meals are countereffective to your muscle. There are two reasons why:

First, exercise causes temporary disruption in glucose utilization in your muscle. That's due to muscle microtrauma (the wear and tear of the muscle tissue). Hence, right after exercise, your muscle can't tolerate high-glycemic meals.

Second, high-glycemic meals impair your insulin, disrupt your muscle mTOR, and shatter your muscle protein synthesis. mTOR is the biological mechanism that builds your muscle, and it can't be fully activated when your insulin is insensitive (see Chapter 2).

Chronic intake of high-glycemic meals has been shown to cause hyperinsulinemia, a condition in which insulin is chronically over-spiked. Hyperinsulinemia has been linked to uncontrollable fat gain as well as irreversible damage to insulin receptors and devastation of the muscular system.

Scientists worldwide agree that the human body hasn't evolved to do well on high-glycemic meals. And there's a strong association between high-glycemic diets and the current epidemics of obesity, diabetes, cardiovascular disease, and cancer.

Let's take a closer look at how your meal's glycemic load affects your muscle.

How Your Meal's Glycemic Load Affects Your Muscle

As noted, after exercise your muscle becomes temporarily insulin resistant. That's due to tissue microinjuries, which impair the mechanism that utilizes glucose in your muscle.

Putting a high-glycemic fuel in your muscle right after exercise can jeopardize its energy utilization. High-glycemic fuels include all sugars, refined flours, and dried fruits.

This doesn't mean that you should avoid carbohydrate foods altogether. Under normal conditions, when your muscle is fully recuperated, it should be quite efficient in utilizing carbohydrates. That's if your carbohydrates are low-glycemic from whole fibrous sources such as legumes, roots, whole grains, quinoa, and corn kernels.

But beware that all carbohydrates can be problematic when consumed in excess.

That's indeed a serious problem today. Carbohydrate consumption per capita in the United States is now greater than ever, and our society has been getting increasingly insulin resistant. The vast majority of Americans over the age of fifty suffer from blood sugar disorders, and the rates of obesity and diabetes today are at an all-time high.

The glycemic load of food is a concern that you can't afford overlooking.

Even if you presently tolerate carbohydrates, there is no guarantee that you'll tolerate them in the future. As you age, you typically lose your insulin sensitivity along with the capacity to utilize carbohydrates for energy. This means that as you get older, you need to put even more attention to the glycemic load of your meals.

To keep your muscle nourished and functional, avoid high-glycemic meals. Avoid candies and stay away from sugar-loaded protein powders and energy bars.

How should you choose your muscle fuel? That's next.

Chapter 18

Your Fuel Choice

Finding the right fuel for your muscle is a must. Your fuel can affect not only how your muscle utilizes energy, but also whether your muscle builds up or breaks down. Inadequate muscle fueling can result in energy crashes, loss of strength, a sluggish metabolism, and undesirable fat gain.

Your muscle can use all food groups as a fuel, but it has its own priorities, and these are dictated by specific needs. There are three fuel options: protein, carbohydrate, and fat. You need to know how to choose between them.

Protein Fuel: Is It Superior or Inferior?

Out of the three fuel foods, protein is the most tricky. It could be your best or worst fuel.

Your body generally uses protein fuel as a last resort. It becomes a primary fuel only when there's a severe energy deficiency, such as due to fasting or intense exhaustive physical drills. Under these conditions, protein becomes a survival fuel, and a most efficient one.

Your body can utilize protein fuel in two ways. It can either break amino acids for immediate energy or use amino acids for glucose synthesis.

The process that converts amino acids to glucose is the most efficient fueling mechanism in your body (see Chapter 1). Called the alanine-glucose cycle, it releases to your muscle exactly the right amount of glucose needed, no more, no less—100 percent efficiency. And all this without raising your insulin or blood sugars.

This primal fueling mechanism seems to serve an important biological purpose. It enabled early humans to endure extreme physical hardship during times of food scarcity and poor accessibility to carbohydrates.

Given this, protein is your best fuel only when your diet is low in carbohydrates. A high-carbohydrate diet will shut down your alanine-glucose cycle and render your protein fuel inefficient.

What's the Downside of Protein Fuel?

When eaten in excess along with a high carbohydrate intake, protein is wasted as inefficient fuel. It isn't a "clean fuel"; protein breaks down into nitrogen metabolites, which need to be neutralized by your liver and kidneys. And even though high protein intake has been shown to be quite safe and cause no kidney disorders in healthy people, it may strain the kidneys of individuals suffering from kidney insufficiencies.

Unlike carbs or fat, protein can't be stored in the muscle as a fuel per se. In order to use protein as a reserve fuel, your body needs to extract it from your muscles.

Does it mean that protein breakdown is bad for your muscle?

Not necessarily. Protein breakdown is actually an essential process that benefits your muscle. Let's see how.

How Protein Breakdown Benefits Your Muscle

Muscle-protein breakdown is a vital metabolic process that plays an important role in recycling your muscle tissues. It involves removal of broken proteins and damaged cells to allow synthesis of new proteins and regeneration of new muscle cells. That's one of the greatest benefits of exercise and fasting: both break and recycle your muscle tissue, keeping it young and viable.

Muscle-protein breakdown becomes an issue only when it chronically surpasses muscle-protein synthesis, such as due to starvation or muscle disease.

Your Fuel Affinity: Carbohydrate versus Fat

Normally, both dietary carbohydrate and dietary fat can be utilized as primary fuels. Nonetheless, people have different affinities for these fuels. Some people do well on carbohydrate fuel, and some do better on fat fuel. And there are those who perform well on both fuels. But there are also people who can't tolerate either. They can't utilize carbohydrates, and they can't metabolize fat.

To understand which fuel works best for you, we need to take a closer look at your muscle-fueling system. How does it operate?

Your Muscle-Fueling System

Your muscle-fueling system is quite picky. It doesn't tolerate a mixed fuel.

When your muscle is fed primarily with carbohydrate fuel, fat-metabolizing enzymes are inhibited. And when your muscle is fed with fat fuel, carbohydrate-metabolizing enzymes are inhibited.

Your muscle prefers to deal with one primary fuel at a time, either carbohydrate, fat, or protein. Proper muscle fueling requires you to always select one kind of primary fuel.

But this doesn't mean that you can't eat protein, fat, and carbs together. It simply means that only one of these fuels can serve as a *primary* fuel.

For instance, if you choose almonds as a primary fat fuel, the naturally occurring carbs in the nut will not be a problem. Similarly, if you choose potatoes as a primary source of carbohydrate fuel, adding a small amount of olive oil on top is OK.

But if you combine large, equal amounts of fat and carbohydrates together, such as by having a bowl of mashed potatoes with a bowl of almonds, the two primary fuels will reject each other. As a result, your muscle's fueling will be compromised, and much of this mix of fuel calories will be converted to triglycerides and body fat rather than energy.

So how do you choose your fuel?

Choosing Your Fuel

Three major factors dictate whether you have an affinity for a certain fuel:

- Your state of health
- Your level of fitness
- Your training protocol

Whatever your condition is at any given time, you need a fuel choice that suits your specific needs.

For instance, if you're healthy, lean, and physically fit, you'll most likely do well on both carb and fat fuels. If, however, you suffer from health issues such as disorders in blood sugar or blood lipids, or if you are excessively overweight, your fuel choice must be carefully adjusted.

- In case of blood-sugar disorders, use protein or fat fuel.
- In case of blood-lipid disorders, use protein or carbohydrate fuel.
- In case of metabolic syndrome (blood-sugar and blood-lipids disorders), use protein fuel.
- In case of obesity, use mostly protein fuel.

Fuel for Your Specific Training

Your fuel choice should accommodate your specific training protocol.

Fuel for Endurance

If you're engaged in endurance drills, use either carbohydrate or fat fuels. Intense endurance works your Type IIA fast muscle fibers, which allow you to use both fuels.

If, however, you're engaged in prolonged endurance training, you can greatly benefit from glycogen loading. For that purpose, carbohydrates should be your first choice. Fat fuel can also be used for glycogen loading, but it will take it a longer time to yield the same effect.

This means that you should schedule your glycogen loading according to your fuel choice. If you choose carbohydrates, start your loading a day before the event. If you choose fat, start your loading two to three days before the event.

Fuel for Weight Lifting

If you're mainly engaged in heavy weight lifting, which works primarily your Type IIB fast muscle fibers, you'll need more carbohydrate fuel, which inherently suits these fibers. And as noted, you can certainly use protein fuel to sustain your strength during prolonged sets.

Fuel for Both Strength and Endurance

If you combine strength and endurance in your exercise regimen, you'll work your Type IIA fast fibers, which means you can use all fuels—carbs, fat, and protein.

But there's another important determinant of your fuel type. That's your level of fitness.

Your Fitness Level and Your Fuel Choice

The fitter you are, the more durable your muscle becomes, and the better you will do on all fuels, but especially fat fuel. Exercise seems to increase mitochondrial size and fat utilization in all muscle fibers. So the more trained your muscle is, the more efficient it will be at utilizing fat fuel.

Cycling between Your Protein, Carb, and Fat Fuels

Even if you find your specific fuel, you should still try to cycle between days of protein, carbs, and fat. Check how the fuel cycle itself affects your energy and performance, and then adjust it accordingly.

The best way to cycle fuels is by incorporating your primary fuel throughout most of the week, and then have your secondary fuel for the remaining days.

For instance, if your primary fuel is carbs, you'll need to incorporate more days of carb fuel than days of protein or fat fuel during the week. And if your primary fuel is fat, incorporate more days of fat fuel than days of protein or carb fuel.

You can design your weekly fuel cycle in any way that works for you. Using primarily carbs fuel, this might mean two days of carbs followed by one day of fat, three days of carbs, and one day of protein. Or it might mean four days of carbs, one day of fat, one day of protein, and another day of fat.

And if you're using primarily fat fuel, the same method should be applied with the fuel priority reversed.

Protein should be your primary fuel only when carbohydrates or fat are not available. Nonetheless, it's worth training your body to handle protein fuel a day at a time.

Try to write down how each fuel cycle affects your energy, performance, and body weight. If you feel that your energy declines, or if you notice an undesirable weight gain, it means that you need to change and adjust your fuel cycle. Over time, this will prove essential in designing your ideal nutritional regimen.

Your Short-Term and Long-Term Muscle Fuels

Your muscle needs both short-term and long-term fuels. Your short-term fast fuel should be used mainly as an instant energy boost such as before and after exercise. Your long-term fuel from slow-assimilating food should be used primarily for long-lasting energy replenishment such as during the night.

> *Short-Term Fuels*
> **Protein:** Whey protein, yogurt, kefir
> **Carbohydrate:** Berries, pomegranates, bananas
> **Fat:** MCT oil from coconut

> *Long-Term Fuels*
> **Protein:** Cheese, eggs, fish, meat, poultry
> **Carbohydrate:** Legumes, roots, whole grains, corn kernels
> **Fat:** Almonds, pistachios, cashews, chia seeds, avocados

Can You Use Syrups as Short-Term Fuels?

All syrups have a relatively high glycemic load and therefore aren't suitable for postexercise recovery. If you choose to use a syrup, it should be applied in very small amounts (no more than a few grams) to avoid glycemic reactions. Your best choices are maple, tapioca, and coconut syrups, which compared to other sugar syrups are lower in fructose as well as glycemic load.

Industrial Fructose: Your Worst Fuel

Your worst fuel is industrial fructose. This commercially processed sugar is commonly found in juices, candies, and food products. It's also a common ingredient in protein shakes, protein bars, diet products, and energy drinks, where it is branded as high-fructose corn syrup or crystalline fructose.

Fructose is low-glycemic but nevertheless toxic. It shatters sugar metabolism by bypassing your body's normal insulin pathway.

After fructose is ingested, your insulin remains nonresponsive and therefore fails to regulate your liver's sugar metabolism. Consequently, sugar metabolites start to accumulate in your liver, which then becomes glucose intolerant. And at this point, a general state of insulin resistance occurs in your body.

Note that your body has a low metabolic threshold for fructose; it tends to convert it to triglycerides and body fat rather than energy. High fructose consumption has been linked to obesity, diabetes, and a host of related disorders.

Fructose is fatal to human health. Even your muscle rejects it. Fructose is now considered one of the major culprits behind the current epidemic of modern human disease.

Next we'll take a look at your meal size and meal timing.

Chapter 19

Your Meal Size

Your meal size determines how efficiently you utilize your food. The smaller your meal is, the better it is utilized by your body. And the same applies for your protein serving: the smaller it is, the more efficiently it is assimilated and utilized.

This means that pound for pound, small protein meals deliver more protein to your muscle than large protein meals do. But then again, even though large protein meals are less efficient, they yet provide more protein to your muscle than small protein meals.

So how do you optimize your small and large protein meals to yield maximum protein utilization efficiency?

Optimizing Your Small Protein Meals

It has been found that the threshold protein needed to grant maximum utilization efficiency is about 20 to 30 g per serving. Anything beyond that will start wasting protein.

Some researchers say that the typical western diet wastes over 60 percent of its protein intake. And the reason for that has to do with wrong meal design. Our meals are generally too big and too frequent, and the body can't make use of all the protein in them. Incredibly, a 30-g protein serving can yield almost the same net protein utilization as a 50-g serving, and with a lower digestive stress and less nitrogen wasted.

To maximize protein deposit in your muscle from your small protein meals, you need to make them with fast-assimilating proteins and incorporate them at a high frequency—every two to three hours. Known as "pulse feeding," this approach grants maximum protein utilization efficiency. Frequent, small protein meals aren't just more effective than the same intake of protein from large meals, they're also easier to digest. And they can benefit athletes as well as ordinary people.

All that said, you can still enjoy eating a large meal and keep a relatively high rate of protein utilization, but you need to know how to design them accordingly.

Optimizing Your Large Protein Meals

To keep a high rate of protein utilization from your large meal, you need to adjust your calorie intake.

Researchers have found that the efficiency of protein utilization increases by sheer calorie intake. So by adding sufficient fuel calories to your large protein meal, you can actually boost its protein utilization rate.

If you like eating larger portions of meat or fish, for instance, you'd need to add additional fuel food to the meal. Hence, meat and potatoes will utilize more protein than the meat alone. And fish with nuts will utilize more protein than fish alone.

For anabolic purposes, a protein should always come with either carbohydrate or fat fuel. And since fat fuel is twice as calorie-dense as carbohydrate fuel, you actually need half the amount of fat than carbohydrates in your meals.

In conclusion, you can benefit from both your small and large protein meals. But you need to know how to time them. Your meal timing is next.

Chapter 20

Your Meal Timing

When you eat makes *what* you eat matters. Even properly designed meals must be eaten at the right time. Otherwise, nutrient delivery will be compromised, and your meal may turn countereffective.

So when is the best time to feed your muscle?

The best time is when your muscle is most recipient to absorb nutrients. There are two such windows of opportunity. The first opportunity is after fasting, and the second is after exercise.

Let's take a closer look at this.

Feeding after Fasting

After fasting, your body is at its highest capacity to digest and utilize food. Your stomach is loaded with digestive enzymes, and your muscle is in a peak anabolic mode to assimilate nutrients and protein. That's a great window of opportunity for feeding your muscle. But there is another bonus involved.

When your stomach's enzyme pool is fully loaded after fasting, protease enzymes reach the circulation where they systematically search for and destroy sick cells and pathogenic elements. Enzyme loading via fasting seems to be a great natural strategy to support the body's defenses and prevent the formation of cancer cells.

Feeding after Exercise

Right after exercise, there is a window of opportunity in which your muscle becomes most receptive to absorbing protein. This is apparently part of a compensation mechanism that promotes muscle recovery after the wear and tear of exercise.

To fully take advantage of that window, you need to feed your muscle with one to three small, low-glycemic, fast-assimilating protein meals. Hence, small whey protein meals.

In practical terms, have your first recovery meal about thirty minutes after exercise and then follow with your second meal about an hour later. Your third recovery meal is optional, and it should be taken an hour or two after your second recovery meal.

The frequent use of small, fast-assimilating protein meals has been shown to be most anabolic. Pound for pound, pulse feeding yields faster and higher protein utilization than any other feeding approach.

But you should never force-feed yourself. For instance, if you feel that one postexercise recovery meal is enough, don't force yourself to eat a second meal.

Again, your recovery meals should be fast assimilating. No matter what your age is, or what shape you're in, your body needs fast nourishment after exercise. Cooked meat, chicken, and fish aren't good choices for postexercise recovery.

All that said, recovery meals have their own limitations. They're good for certain purposes, but you can't live on them alone.

Your body requires both fast- and slow-assimilating foods. Fast-assimilating meals serve to instantly support your muscle, whereas slow-assimilating meals offer you longer-lasting nourishment, greater protein intake, and greater energy replenishment.

So when is the right time to eat these two types of meal?

Timing Your Meals around Your Innate Circadian Clock

You need to time your meals according to your innate circadian clock which is programmed in your autonomic nervous system (ANS). The autonomic nervous system regulates all your activities throughout the day and night. It is divided into two parts: a daily one and a nightly one.

During the day, you're under the control of the sympathetic nervous system (SNS). The SNS is responsible for keeping you awake, alert, and active, and it encourages your body to resist fatigue, spend energy, and burn fat.

But your SNS is highly sensitive to your feeding status.

It is actually stimulated by lack of food and suppressed by large meals. Your SNS can only tolerate foods that are light and low-glycemic, such as light proteins, whole fruits, and vegetables. And every time you eat a large or high-glycemic meal, you shut your SNS down.

Instead, you turn on your nightly nervous system—the parasympathetic nervous system (PSNS). The PSNS makes you tired, sluggish, and ready to go to sleep, and it suppresses fat burning. That's why you typically feel tired and sleepy after a big lunch.

Nonetheless, the PSNS enhances your digestion and promotes the replenishment of nutrients and energy.

So how do you time your meals?

Timing Your Small Meals

Your small protein meals should be incorporated during daytime. This allows you to stay alert, focused, and active during the working hours of the day, and you can actually nourish your muscle and burn fat at the same time.

Start your day with a mix of your favorite fast-assimilating protein, optionally with whole fruits or vegetable juices. Having whey protein with blueberries or carrot juice, for instance, is a great way to jump-start your day. This will nourish your muscle while keeping your SNS intact. Eating small servings of yogurt, fresh cheese, or eggs with whole fruits or a green salad is also a viable option. You can have your small muscle meals (20 to 30 g protein per serving) every few hours.

But remember to allow a sufficient break between your meals for complete digestion and better utilization of nutrients.

Timing Your Large Meals

Your large meals should contain both raw and cooked food and should be made with denser and slow-digesting foods. The best time for such meals is the evening—yes, contrary to common opinion.

Technically, during the evening your body is under the control of the PSNS, which promotes relaxation and enhances your digestion. Night is indeed your right time to calm down, digest food, and replenish energy.

Humans evolved to be nocturnal eaters. Your autonomic nervous system and your innate circadian clock bear proof of that. In ancient societies, supper was the main and often the only meal of the day. You utilize meals better at nighttime when you are at rest. And you don't digest well during the daytime when you are under stress.

Animal studies revealed that consuming one main meal per day or every other day, yields outstanding health benefits. These include protection against diabetes and neurodegenerative disease, as well as improved body composition and a substantial increase in life span. (We'll look at this in more detail later on.)

At night, you can choose from a large variety of whole protein foods including wild-catch fish, organic eggs, organic dairy, free-range chicken, or grass-fed animals' meat. However, try one protein source at a time, and see how it works for you.

Your fuel foods should come from either raw nuts and seeds or from whole unrefined carbohydrate foods. But remember, don't combine these two types of fuel foods at the same meal (except for legumes, which can be mixed with fat fuel).

And most importantly, try to increase your intake of vegetables in your evening meal, both raw and cooked. Fruit and vegetables are your primary antioxidant foods. And as we'll see next, they're most crucial for your muscle's sustainability and buildup.

Chapter 21

Your Antioxidant Foods

Your antioxidant intake is crucial. It affects how your body resists oxidative stress and reflects how your muscle resists degradation. Exercise causes accumulation of oxidative stress in your muscle, and you need to counteract this with sufficient intake of antioxidants.

Your muscle is inherently equipped to defend itself with its own antioxidant proteins and enzymes, but these must be enhanced by dietary antioxidants and immunosupportive nutrients. And since the typical diet often fails to support your body's antioxidant requirements, you need to incorporate a special nutritional strategy for granting sufficient antioxidant intake.

Deficiencies of vitamins, minerals, and antioxidants are highly prevalent today, particularly among athletes. Such deficiencies occur even if the diet itself provides the minimum recommended daily allowance of essential nutrients.

So what can you do to enhance your antioxidant defenses?

First, you need to increase your intake of antioxidant foods. These include fresh fruits, vegetables, nuts, seeds, roots, and spices such as turmeric, cumin, oregano, thyme, and all caffeinated teas (black and green). Two of the most powerful foods in this category are dark chocolate and quality whey protein. Combining dark chocolate with whey protein may be your best bet.

Both chocolate and whey are classified as super foods. Dark chocolate is exceptionally high in antioxidant polyphenols, known for their neuroprotective and metabolic-supportive properties. Quality whey is known for its outstanding immune-boosting, muscle-nourishing properties. Quality dark chocolate and whey protein yield a most powerful super food blend with unmatched nutritional value.

Let's take a look at how food's antioxidant capacity is measured.

Oxygen Radical Absorbance Capacity (ORAC)

Oxygen radical absorbance capacity (ORAC) indicates how well a certain food can absorb oxidative radicals. Foods with high ORAC scores are known to be most beneficial in preventing cellular oxidative damage. High-ORAC foods serve best at fighting disease, tissue degradation, and aging.

Foods with the highest ORAC scores include dark chocolate, teas, stabilized rice germ, blueberries, raspberries, pomegranate, and acai and goji berries. Other notably high-ORAC foods include cilantro, parsley, papaya, mango, pepper, citrus, onion, cooked tomatoes, grasses, and all leafy green vegetables.

Keep Your Diet Clean

Along with the consumption of high-ORAC antioxidant foods, it's important to keep your diet clean from chemical toxins, rancid food, damaged protein, artificial additives, sugar alcohol, yeast extract, refined starches, sugar, and fructose. All these are harmful substances that deplete your body's antioxidant reserves.

Antioxidant Foods

The following chart features a list of common antioxidant foods, with their respected properties:

Food Type	Examples	Benefits
Green vegetables	Parsley, cilantro, leafy greens, and grasses	Provide the largest range of water-soluble antioxidants and beneficial saccharides along with fat-soluble antioxidants and essential nutrients, including vitamin C and bioflavonoids, B vitamins, vitamin K, pro-vitamin A, minerals, and chlorophyll, known for their antioxidant, detoxifying, anti-inflammatory, and healing properties.
Yellow, orange, and red vegetables, roots, and fruits	Carrot, pepper, yam, pumpkin, squash tomato, papaya, melon	Provide fat-soluble, pro-vitamin A antioxidants, including, beta-carotene, lycopene, and lutein, known for their antioxidant, immunosupportive properties and protection against ultraviolet radiation (UV). Beta-carotene works as a cofactor in recycling vitamin E.
	Onion, garlic	Provide rich amounts of immuno-supportive, antioxidant, anti-inflammatory antibiotic nutrients.
Cruciferous vegetables	Broccoli, cauliflower, cabbage, brussels sprouts	Provide sulfur-rich phytonutrients and indoles, known for their antioxidant, anticarcinogenic, and hormonal-supportive properties.
Raw nuts and seeds	Almonds, pistachios, cashews, pecans, walnuts, chia seeds, pumpkin seeds	Provide significant amounts of fat-soluble antioxidants, vitamin E tocopherols and tocotrienols, minerals, and phytonutrient cofactors for preventing cellular lipid peroxidation and damage to the mitochondria. Rich sources of essential oils and metabolic supportive phytosterols.

Food Type	Examples	Benefits
All fruits	Blueberries, raspberries, blackberries, mulberries, strawberries, amla berries, goji berries, acai berries, figs, kiwis, pomegranate, apples, citrus fruits, black currant, papayas, mangos, and melons	Provide water-soluble antioxidants including vitamins, flavonoid polyphenols, flavonones, tannins, and terpenoid glycocides, all of which are potent free-radical-scavenging, anticarcinogenic, and immune-boosting nutrients. Berries are the most nutrient-dense among all fruits. Pomegranate, figs, citrus, kiwis, and papayas are also great sources of antioxidant, immunosupportive, and anticarcinogenic phytonutrients.
Whey protein	Grass-fed cows' whey protein—cold processed from raw milk with no sugar added, no sugar alcohol, no fructose, and no chemical additives	Richest source of fragile amino acids (commonly missing in the diet), immunoglobulins, antioxidant peptides, and CLA, known for their immune-protective, metabolic-supportive, and anti-aging properties. The naturally occurring cysteine in whey has been shown to boost the body's master antioxidant glutathione, along with its antioxidant enzymes.
Dark chocolate	Premium dark chocolate, alkali-free with no sugar added, no sugar alcohol, no fructose, and no chemical additives	Richest source of antioxidant polyphenols with the highest lipophilic ORAC among all foods. Dark chocolate has outstanding lneuro-protective and muscle-supportive properties. It has been shown to support muscle recovery better than sport drinks of the same amount of calories.

You need to cover your antioxidant bases and support your body's defenses every day; that's including in times of limited accessibility to antioxidant food. For that purpose you may need to use nutritional supplements. But you need to be careful with your choices ...

Some of these products may actually cause more harm than benefit.

Which supplements will benefit you and which may harm you? That's next.

Chapter 22

Your Antioxidant Supplements

It has been widely known that antioxidant supplementation helps decrease oxidative damage in the body. Studies indicate that antioxidant supplementation helps boost energy and reduce muscle fatigue.

But there are also contradictory reports regarding antioxidant supplements, particularly regarding the use of synthetic antioxidants.

There's a difference between natural and synthetic supplements. Natural supplements are food based, whereas synthetic supplements are chemical based.

So how do natural antioxidant supplements benefit your muscle? What are your best choices in this category? And what supplements should you beware of?

How Natural Antioxidants Benefit Your Muscle

Recent studies have indicated that natural antioxidant supplements, such as natural vitamin E and C, attenuate lipid peroxidation and energy decline in the muscle during exercise. These supplements have also been shown to reduce muscle inflammation.

Inflammation is one of the leading causes of oxidative damage in the muscle. When inflammation becomes chronic, muscle fibers are damaged by accumulated free radicals, and the muscle is rendered dysfunctional. To counteract muscle inflammation, you need to increase your intake of antioxidant nutrients.

In theory, you should be able to get all the key nutrients you need from food alone. But due to soil depletion and modern industrial processing, grocery food is largely deficient in essential nutrients. Consequently, the typical diet fails to fully support your physical needs.

In today's world, antioxidant supplementation is important. And it's becoming more crucial when your body is under increased oxidative stress such as due to intense physical training, injury, disease, or aging.

But not all antioxidant supplements are the same. Some supplements may cause more harmful effects than benefits.

Harmful Antioxidants: How Synthetic Antioxidants Impair Your Muscle and Health

It has been largely assumed that antioxidant supplementation can help protect against oxidative damage. However, while this seems correct, in real life it isn't always true.

Researchers have been finding growing evidence that synthetic antioxidants actually cause more harm than benefit to the body and particularly the muscle. Ironically, these are the most prevalent and most medically endorsed products today.

So how do synthetic antioxidants harm your muscle?

It seems that a certain threshold of oxidative stress is necessary to keep your muscle tuned. And that threshold is characterized by low levels of free radicals. You see, free radicals are to your muscle like mice to a cat: they keep your muscle alert and ready for action.

Emerging evidence indicates that high dosages of synthetic antioxidants such as synthetic vitamin C ascorbate, vitamin E, or Ubiquinol disrupt and decrease muscle performance. Synthetic antioxidants have been shown to impair muscle contractibility and decrease its strength, speed, and durability.

Studies on greyhound race dogs have shown that synthetic vitamin C administration caused the animals to lose 30 percent of their initial speed. And human studies have been showing that synthetic antioxidants impair muscle adaptability to exercise.

The supplements industry may tell the opposite, but the evidence is undeniable. The human body has never adapted to do well on antioxidant megadosages. Your body is not programmed to accept synthetic supplements, and you should only support your body with food-based antioxidants.

Recommended Antioxidant Supplements

Following is a range of recommended antioxidant supplements. Your choices and dosages depend on your particular needs and level of activity:

Plant-Based Multivitamins and Minerals

Your body evolved to depend exclusively on essential nutrients from food. Make sure that your vitamin product is all natural and food-based, with no synthetic or yeast-based ingredients added.

Amla C/Natural Vitamin C

Vitamin C plays a number of essential roles in your body. In addition to being an antioxidant, vitamin C is a catalyst in the production of your brain's neurotransmitters dopamine and adrenaline. It also assists in the synthesis of the amino acid carnitine, which plays a key role in your muscle's fat fuel utilization.

Furthermore, vitamin C is vital for tissue maintenance. Your body uses it for the buildup of collagen, a protein component essential for the formation and restoration of your connective tissues.

Vitamin C must be taken in its natural form, as it naturally occurs in plants, together with its bioflavonoids and cofactors.

The best natural source of vitamin C is amla berries. Other great natural sources are citrus fruits and peels, blueberries, raspberries, blackberries, strawberries, goji berries, acai, kiwis, and peppers. Amla C is now available in supplement form.

Beware of Yeast-Based Supplements

Some of the most popular natural supplements today are made from yeast. And even though labeled as 100-percent natural, these products aren't really food-based.

Yeast has never been used traditionally as a viable food for humans. It's highly allergenic, and its processing yields a dangerous neurotoxic by-product of yeast fermentation called monosodium glutamate (MSG). Some reports indicate that all kinds of dietary yeast present a health risk and therefore should be avoided.

The safest and most viable source of vitamins and antioxidant nutrients are plants. Plant food and plant-based supplements in the form of botanical extracts, teas, and potions have been used traditionally for thousands of years to support human health.

Herbal Antioxidants and Detoxifiers

The following list of herbs (some of which you might recognize as spices) have been used traditionally for toning, cleansing, and healing purposes.

Toning, Cleansing, and Healing Herbs

Shilajit asphaltum *General tonic, anti-inflammatory recovery agent, potency enhancer*	Oregano *Antioxidant, antimicrobial, antiseptic digestive aid, sedative*	Embilica fruit (Amla C) *Vitamin C complex, antioxidant, anti-inflammatory, healing aid adrenal supportive, anticancer*	Ashwagandha root *Adaptogen, cognitive aid, sedative and ergogenic, anti-inflammatory, anticancer*
Apigenin *Antioxidant, antibacterial, hormonal supportive, sedative, skin aid*	Thyme *Antiseptic, respiratory aid, antioxidant*	Triphala fruit *Cleansing and digestive aid, digestive aid, blood purifier*	Ginger root *Stimulant, digestive and nausea-relieving aid, metabolic supportive*

Toning, Cleansing, and Healing Herbs (continued)

Resveratrol *Antioxidant, antibacterial, antifungal, metabolic supportive, anticancer*	Turmeric *Antibacterial, anti-inflammatory, antioxidant, neuro-rejuvenator, hormonal supportive, anticancer*	Bacopa leaves *Neuro-protective brain herb, adaptogen, metabolic supportive, ergogenic*	Dandelion root *Anti-inflammatory, liver and kidney cleansing aid, diuretic*
Pycnogenol (Pine bark extract) *Antioxidant, metabolic supportive*	Cardamom fruit *Antibacterial, kidney cleanser, digestive aid, anti-inflammatory*	Milk thistle seeds *Liver cleanser and rejuvenator, antioxidant, anticancer, immune enhancer*	Boerhavia root *Blood purifier, anti-inflammatory, detoxifier*

Some additional notes on traditional herbs:

- Shilajit has been regarded by Ayurvedic, Chinese, and Russian physicians as the panacea for healing and tissue rejuvenation. It has been successfully used to balance blood sugar, alleviate kidney or liver insufficiencies, treat injuries, enhance libido, and support muscle recovery.
- Turmeric's active ingredient curcumin has been shown to increase the levels of brain-derived neurotrophic factor (BDNF). BDNF plays key neuro-protective roles, activating stem cells to regenerate new brain neurons. It has been shown to counteract stress-related depression, improve long-term memory, and enhance cognitive function. BDNF is also expressed in other tissues including neuro-motors, the kidneys, and the prostate. Low levels of BDNF have been linked to depression, schizophrenia, obsessive-compulsive disorder, anorexia nervosa, Alzheimer's disease, and dementia.
- While not antioxidants per se, probiotics—your beneficial gut bacteria—are essential for your health. These friendly bacteria

protect your digestive tract from pathogenic yeast colonization, and they finalize the digestion and utilization of protein. Probiotics increase the biological value of proteins. They also play an important role in the elimination of waste toxins. Probiotics are available in the form of special yogurts or pills.

Your Antioxidant Defenses in Summary

Your body's first line of antioxidant defense should come from whole plant foods, including fresh vegetables, fruits, roots, nuts, seeds, spices, and chocolate. Dark chocolate is a most potent antioxidant superfood, and even more so when combined with quality whey protein.

Your body's second line of antioxidant defense should come from natural food-based supplements. These include plant-based vitamins and minerals as well as immunosupportive and cleansing herbal formulas.

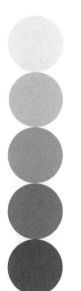

PART IV

Discussion

Chapter 23

Your Muscle and Longevity

The dream of eternal life has been inherent to human cultures since the dawn of civilization. It should come as no surprise that scientists have taken up the challenge to search for a biological switch that will turn off the aging process. The first evidence that such a switch exists emerged about seventy years ago when researchers found that mice given extremely minimal calories were consistently living longer than normal. Incredibly, they lived as much as 40 percent longer.

The notion that calorie restriction can increase life span has since been controversial and highly arguable. Can we accept the idea that near starvation is healthy?

We habitually like eating lots of food all day long, and most of us will fail to restrict calorie intake even if trying to. So here we are today desperate for something else—something that can extend life but requires no calorie restriction and no hustle.

The Longevity Pill

According to recent news reports, researchers have managed to identify the first longevity gene. That's apparently the gene linked to calorie restriction.

Not surprisingly, these findings have opened the door for commercial interests and a great deal of speculation. The very possibility of developing a pill that works like calorie restriction and allows people to stop aging regardless of how they eat or live seems like a dream come true.

One of the first substances proposed to fit this bill is a compound called resveratrol. In its natural form, resveratrol is an antioxidant, antifungal phytonutrient found in grape skin, raspberries, mulberries, and red wine.

Nonetheless, the so-called longevity pill on the market is actually made from synthetic resveratrol (you can't patent and profit from natural food ingredients). The company behind this drug claims that it triggers the same longevity gene as calorie restriction. But will it be that miracle pill? And will it stop you from aging?

Could You Stop Aging by Popping a Pill?

Longevity is inherent to your body. It's essentially triggered by how you eat, exercise, and live. There is no pill in the world that will ever change that. No pill will ever substitute the effects of exercise, fasting, and good nutrition on your genes.

And even if scientists will figure out a way to genetically modify your body for living longer, it will most likely come as a trade-off—you'll need to give up on something in return. But at what price?

Anti-Aging in Practice

A real longevity impact requires the full activation of your anti-aging apparatus.

Your body doesn't want to fail; nor does it want to get sick or overweight. And it certainly doesn't want to die. Quite the opposite. Your body is well programmed to thrive. It's by all means capable of sustaining and rejuvenating itself. Wounds can heal themselves; skin can be restored; and bones can be rebuilt. And the muscle is no different.

When your longevity genes are triggered, they activate mechanisms that improve your energy efficiency, recycle old and damaged cells, and rejuvenate your tissues. Your body not only retains its youthful appearance, it also gets stronger and healthier. And you'll be able to enjoy living longer.

But how do you trigger your longevity genes? And what shuts them down?

Your Longevity Apparatus

In reality, many genes and pathways have been found to govern the aging process in your body. These are cross-linked, and their combined anti-aging effect is highly complex to say the least.

Two of the most notable metabolic pathways that affect your longevity are the *insulin/IGF signaling pathway* and the *mitochondrial electron transport chain pathway* (the mitochondrial energy system). These critical pathways are linked to your muscle. They regulate sustainability, growth, and energy utilization in your body. And the key for unlocking the anti-aging process in your body is in the very genes that preserve these pathways.

Other longevity genes are those encoding brain neurotrophins, muscle myogenic regulatory factors (MRFs), and other tissue-specific growth factors that activate stem and satellite cells to commit and differentiate into new cells and regenerate new tissues.

What Triggers Your Longevity Genes?

Your body thrives when under nutritional and physical stress. Both calorie restriction and physical hardship are perceived by your body as survival signals to adapt and improve.

The effects of calorie restriction and physical hardship on your longevity seem to be deeply rooted in your biology. Both trigger biological mechanisms that evolved to help humans endure times of food scarcity and extreme physical hardship.

These primal biological mechanisms are part of your survival system. They have been essential for keeping our species alive for as long as we've been on this planet. When triggered, these mechanisms compensate your body by protecting your insulin system, strengthening your immune defenses, recycling your tissues, and upgrading your muscle fiber quality.

Survival, it seems, requires stress and action. And action rejects aging. To trigger your longevity genes, you need to routinely challenge your body. You need to train and feed your body as it was originally destined.

It has been widely agreed among scientists that the human body is not programmed for a world of plenty. Your body declines and deteriorates from chronic indulgence and lack of challenge.

But we live today in a world that constantly inundates us with indulgence, and we pay the consequences of that.

We're Shifting Away from Our Species' Original Program

Our society is largely accustomed to technical solutions; there's this common belief in the ultimate power of technology to fix virtually everything.

People want to believe that there's a technical solution to aging. They want to believe that once that magic formula for stopping aging is found, it will be available in the form of a pill at the neighborhood pharmacy.

It seems that almost everything else has been technically simplified, solved, and fixed. Nowadays, we don't need to hunt, fight, or flee to survive. And we hardly ever need to endure hunger, cold, or fear. Virtually everything that early humans had to struggle for is now easily accessible to us.

We have been shifting away from our species' original program and away from the necessity to actively survive. Consequently, we're getting fatter and sicker than ever with soaring rates of obesity, diabetes, cardiovascular disease, and cancer. And if that's not enough, we're also plagued by increasing rates of sterility. Perhaps we're already showing the first signs of species extinction.

And all this relates to one single factor: the denial of our survival code.

The Limitations of Science

It may take many decades for scientists to fully figure out what triggers longevity—if they ever will. Meanwhile, we can't afford to do nothing.

But what can we do without reliable science and viable information?

Science, for all its wonders, has obvious limitations. One of them is the incorporation of studies that investigate isolated factors. That approach often fails to represent real-life conditions and hence fails to yield reliable information.

In the case of muscle conditioning and anti-aging, studies have been commonly investigating isolated factors rather than complex factors. Isolated factors could be, for instance, a specific exercise, a specific nutrient, or a specific supplement. Researchers have been examining how each single factor affects the muscle, or the body, or even the aging process, and the findings get published in prestigious science journals.

But quite often they're of no practical use.

In reality, there are no isolated factors, only complex factors. And our lives aren't running in lab conditions. By investigating only one factor at a time, science has been failing to provide true indications of how things work in real life.

And there is another concern with modern science: animal studies.

Even setting aside the animal cruelty issue, which is largely overlooked, there's also the concern that animals have different metabolisms from humans. Indeed, animal studies often produce results that are different from those expected in human subjects.

For instance, it has been found that high levels of insulin-like growth factor-1 (IGF-1) shorten the life span of mice. In humans, however, high IGF-1 levels are actually linked to an increased life span.

Similarly, recent genetic modification experiments indicated opposite effects on mice and men. Harvard scientists reported a reversal of aging in mice after a certain procedure that reactivates their telomerase enzyme. The telomerase enzyme targets mice's chromosomes to promote cellular division and repair of damaged tissues. However, that same procedure in humans has been known to promote cancer. Apparently, the telomerase enzyme is switched off in adult humans as an evolutionarily protective trait that stops cells from growing out of control and turning into cancer.

Put simply, what extends a rodent's life may actually shorten human life and vice versa. We're not animals, and we should be more cautious when attempting to apply the results of animal studies to ourselves.

Your Muscle and Longevity

Your muscle and longevity are bound together. The genes that sustain and build your muscle are also the genes that extend your life. They're responsible for keeping your energy, cells, and tissues intact.

Your body is programmed to thrive when physically challenged. But your training must accommodate your original makeup.

Based on evolutionary biology, the human body is made with the distinct features of a pack hunter and ambush predator combined. You need to train your body accordingly. That's part of your survival code.

But this doesn't mean that you need to get violent.

Humans are the only predator species that has a choice. You can train aggressively, but you don't need to get violent—unless you're confronted with a threat that leaves you with no other option. Humans evolved to thrive without the necessity to kill (we'll discuss this more in the next chapter).

But you have to practice your survival code. You need to channel your aggression and train in a way that mimics your inherent fight-or-flight program.

Every species has its own survival code along with a distinct fight-or-flight program. Each species spontaneously puts its survival code into practice from birth.

For instance, dog and wolf pups practice nipping, biting, and chasing, learning from their mothers how to pursue a prey and become adult pack hunters. Similarly, kittens and lion cubs practice grappling, striking, and sneak attacking, acquiring from their mothers the skill to become ambush predators.

We're the only species that fails to practice its original survival program.

We typically choose to overlook our predatory nature, though ironically we can't deny who we are. Humans have been fascinated by predatory actions. We love watching predatory events in the form of sport or entertainment. Our society adores boxing, mixed martial arts, and wrestling, and we generally like action movies, but most of us refrain from practicing these types of activities. We typically prefer watching rather than engaging.

Most of us choose pills over actions. It's normal today to be pill dependent and physically inactive. Our longevity genes remain largely dormant, and we gradually lose our ability to survive independently.

Quite often, those who are physically active aren't fully aware of what they're doing. People who exercise regularly are still bouting with weight management and other modern human ailments. Just go to your neighborhood gym and see for yourself. You'll notice that most participants in gym classes are out of shape, and they'll probably look the same or even worse as time goes by . . .

There always seems to be something missing or something wrong with modern fitness. It's lacking solid principles and offers no clear direction.

Even if your exercise choice is adequate, there is no guarantee that your fitness is OK. For instance, strength training typically suppresses durability, whereas endurance training typically suppresses strength. But you need both to be biologically fit. You need to develop special durability along with your strength, all in one cohesive package. That's the way you're programmed to better survive.

It all comes down to one question: *Are you biologically fit?*

Is your muscular system adept at enduring intense, complex hardship? And can you survive independently without drugs and pills? If the answer is Yes and Yes, there is a good chance you'll enjoy longevity.

But your physical conditioning is only one part of the equation. The other part is your nutrition.

Your nutrition and longevity are next.

Chapter 24

Your Nutrition and Longevity

Despite rapidly accumulating data on human nutrition, there has been great confusion as to what diet benefits humans most. To address this issue properly, we need to look into evolutionary biology again. Like other species, we're originally programmed to benefit from specific foods. These foods were part of the early human diet, and as such they fit our biological needs most.

So what is the origin of the human diet? And to what food are we biologically aligned?

What's the Origin of the Human Diet?

Based on fossil evidence, physical anthropology points to several features that distinguished the evolution of humans from other apes. These evolutionary features give us a great indication as to what our original diet was. And they tell us what makes our diet different from that of other apes.

It has been largely agreed that human bipedalism (walking on two legs) is an evolutionary trait that took place before the early Pleistocene (1.75 million years ago). With it came a substantial increase in brain size and a decrease in anterior teeth and jaw size.

The evolution of the human jaw and teeth seems to comprise a functional purpose: adaptation to a specific diet.

According to Clifford J. Jolly, author of *The Seed Eaters*, we have not evolved to eat plant shoots or animal flesh as our primary staple foods.

Human molars and jaw actions are clearly not adapted to mincing grass blades; nor are they adapted to tearing meat apart. Our teeth and jaws are structured to break up small, hard, solid objects that are more or less spherical in shape. This is done by a combination of crushing and rolling such as is employed in milling machines.

Jolly argues that out of potential foods that fit that description, only those that were widespread enough in open country (which was the main human habitat) could serve as the original staple food of humans. These are the seeds of grasses and annual herbs.

That's the premise of Jolly's hypothesis.

However, the idea that the early human's main staple food was seeds alone is highly arguable. Since early humans' main habitat also included woodlands, it's more plausible that the early human diet consisted of both grassland seeds and tree nuts.

The mixed seeds and nuts diet yields a superior protein composition and a higher biological value than a diet based on seeds alone. Hence, a mixed seed-nut diet could have supported human survival better than a seed diet alone.

But there are also logistic reasons why mixed seeds and nuts constituted our original diet. Seeds and nuts offer a larger variety of rancidity-resilient items as compared to seeds alone or animal foods alone. Tree nuts, seeds of tubers, and bulbs are quite resilient to rancidity and could therefore be stored and used all year round. That's unlike meat, sprouted grass grains, or sprouted legume seeds, which are much more perishable and therefore could not be stored and used all year round.

Seeds and nuts seem to define the character of the early human diet. This means that our original diet was primarily low-glycemic, high in fat, and fibrous.

This is not to say that other food resources such as dairy, fish, or meat were not exploited when available. What it indicates is that the early human diet was centered on seeds and nuts. The seed-nut diet has kept humans alive in times when animal food was not accessible, providing sufficient protein, essential nutrients, and fuel calories to sustain life.

Our adaptation to seed-nut chewing is mostly reflected in the flat wear-plane of our cheek teeth. We're the only mammal predator that possess this unique chewing feature. Put simply, we are primarily seed and nut eaters, and we're also capable of eating animal food.

And note that the human diet differs from the chimpanzees' diet, which is mostly based on fruit, and the gorillas' diet, which is largely based on herbage.

So what does that tell us?

Biologically, We're More Gatherers than Hunters

We can eat animal flesh, but we can't depend on it as a main staple food. Meat is not essential to us, but plant foods are.

We can't live on meat alone, and we can't live on fruits alone. But we can live on a seed-nut vegetarian diet, and we can further improve that diet by adding animal food to the mix. The human body is apparently more vegetarian than carnivorous.

We get most of our vital nutrients, vitamins, and antioxidants from plant sources. And unlike other predators such as canines and felines, we're capable of enzymatically utilizing essential oils from plants. We have enzymes (desaturase) that convert plants' long-chain polyunsaturated essential fatty acids into their bioactive forms, EPA, DHA, and GLA.

All that said, our early ancestors were partly carnivorous, and meat cutting was done with tools instead of teeth. We can certainly benefit from animal and marine foods as quality protein sources. Whey protein, cheese, eggs, fish, seafood, and meat have a higher amino acid score than plant food. animal-flesh and marine foods provide unique muscle-supportive compounds, such as beta-alanine and carnosine, that are not found in plant foods. And in this respect they provide superior nourishment to the muscle.

The combination of seeds and nuts with animal or marine food yields ideal nourishment and seems to be a primal fit for our gatherer-hunter nature.

Combining Seeds and Nuts with Animal or Marine Food

Seeds, nuts, and animal or marine foods are complementary food sources that enhance each other's biological value. Animal and marine foods provide quality protein whereas seeds and nuts provide additional protein, essential nutrients, and fuel calories. Combinations of meat, fish, or dairy with seeds or nuts have been used by traditional cuisines around the world, including Mediterranean, Middle Eastern, Indian, and Chinese.

Note that certain varieties of seeds, nuts, animal foods, and marine foods may cause allergic reactions in some people. Make sure that your food selection doesn't include items you're sensitive to.

Before finalizing this topic, we need to address two more issues.

Are we originally programmed to consume carbohydrate food? And how well are we adapted to consume legumes?

Are We Programmed to Consume Grains?

There is a high likelihood that early humans consumed sprouted grains (starch-seeds), which were abundant in open grassland. Nonetheless, grains could not have been the early humans' main staple food for two reasons.

First, unless sprouted, grains are virtually inedible in their raw state. The biological value of grains actually increases upon roasting or baking, and these methods were not used during the early Pleistocene, when the first recognizably human-like evidence appears in the fossil record.

Second, preagricultural grass grains could not provide sufficient protein to support human survival as a main staple food. About five thousand years ago (the beginning of the agricultural era) there was a notable shift in the human diet toward grains. Since then we have been continuously shifting away from our original low-glycemic diet of nuts and seeds toward a diet based on high-glycemic refined carbohydrates, which we are not evolutionarily adapted to.

Are We Programmed to Consume Legumes?

Legumes were available seasonally in open grassland. Grindstones with adherent legume-seed starch appear in the African fossil record. Legumes have the highest protein content among seeds, and that trait could have potentially made them suitable to serve as a main staple food for early humans.

Nonetheless, unless sprouted, soaked, or cooked, legumes contain inhibitors and digestion-disrupting elements that render them problematic for human consumption. It's plausible that humans were gathering young pea pods and sprouted beans seasonally, but the earliest record of legume usage as a main human food appears at about the same time as that of grains. It has been largely agreed that our early ancestors ate every nontoxic seed present in the environment. Whether legume seeds belong to this category remains open to speculation.

But food is only one determining factor in your diet. Other factors are your calorie intake and your meal frequency.

Let's take a look at how these dietary factors affect your health and longevity.

Your Calorie Intake and Longevity

The relation between calorie intake and human longevity has been a subject of great scientific interest.

Based on animal studies, the most proven approach to counteracting aging is calorie restriction. Aside from genetic manipulation, calorie restriction represents the only proven record for prolonging life in animals. And that's not its only benefit.

Tests conducted on laboratory animals have shown that calorie restriction can lower the risk of cancer, diabetes, and cardiovascular disease. It had also been shown to stave off age-related neurodegeneration.

In practice, calorie restriction means lowering normal calorie intake by about 40 to 60 percent. But you still need to maintain a healthy diet rich in vitamins, minerals, and antioxidants. A growing number of people are now living by this regimen. Many of them are scholars and researchers, passionate in their belief that the methodical restriction of their calorie intake can extend their lives.

Can calorie restriction promote longevity in humans? It certainly seems so, but it's still too early to predict. And even if calorie restriction extends life, at what price does it come?

One notable side effect of chronic calorie restriction is the lowering of the body's temperature and metabolic rate. That side effect is essentially an energy-preservation mechanism, and it kicks in when the body's energy intake is chronically low. The consequences of that may include hormonal decline, with decreased thyroid activity and a decline in sex hormones. Metabolic declines of this type have been also associated with loss of muscle strength and libido.

Again, it's still too early to predict, but even if calorie restriction enables people to live longer, it may come at the cost of some of the most important things that make life worth living.

Is there anything else that can be done to trigger your longevity genes, apart from chronically restricting your calorie intake?

Apparently there is one dietary option: intermittent fasting.

Intermittent Fasting: How Meal Frequency Affects Your Longevity

Recent studies have indicated that lowering your meal frequency to one meal per day or every other day may actually provide you with the same benefits as calorie restriction but without restricting your calories.

The initial studies were done on mice. The mice had to go through a special feeding cycle called intermittent fasting, which consisted of a fasting day followed by an overfeeding day in which the mice were allowed to consume twice their normal calorie intake.

The results revealed astonishing longevity benefits. Mice on intermittent fasting have been shown to improve their insulin sensitivity, rejuvenate their brain cells, and substantially increase their life span.

Most importantly, the studies' findings supported the hypothesis that humans and animals evolved to better survive when there's a large gap between meals (at times twenty-four or even forty-eight hours).

According to Dr. Mark Mattson, professor of neurosciences at Johns Hopkins University, humans adapted early on to intermittent fasting as an evolutionary favorite feeding cycle. Mattson, who conducted the initial studies on intermittent fasting, argues that primordial conditions of food scarcity and a hunter-gatherer lifestyle created the necessity to adapt to one meal per day or even every other day.

One of the greatest advantages of intermittent fasting is the rejuvenating impact on your brain and muscle. It literally forces your body to recycle and rejuvenate brain and muscle tissues. Fasting increases the expression of brain-derived neurotrophic factor (BDNF) in your brain and muscle. This neurotrophic growth factor has been shown to catalyze conversion of brain stem cells and muscle satellite cells into new neurons and new muscle cells, respectively. BDNF has profound neuro-protective properties. It plays important roles in brain cognitive function and long-term memory and protects against dementia, Alzheimer's disease, Parkinson's disease, and brain aging. And in addition to this, it also acts on the neuromuscular system, where it protects neuro-motors from degradation and aging.

The rejuvenating effect of fasting on your brain and muscle tissues is more profound than was initially thought.

In your muscle, fasting triggers the removal and recycling of broken proteins and damaged cells. This recycling process is done by the ubiquitin enzymes (your body's demolition force), which detect and digest broken proteins and damaged cells. The nitrogen amino by-products are then recycled and used for synthesis of new proteins and generation of new cells.

Note that this tissue-rejuvenating process is triggered by the catabolic process of protein breakdown such as that due to fasting, exercise, or injury.

Now that we've seen how fasting affects your body, let's take a look at the overfeeding/ compensation phase of intermittent fasting.

During the overfeeding phase, your body shifts from a catabolic recycling mode into an anabolic tissue-building mode. Overfeeding may yield additional benefits. When done properly, it boosts your thyroid and sex hormones along with your body's metabolic rate. And note that if you add a viable exercise protocol to this regimen, it may yield an even stronger impact on your body composition, tissue integrity, and biological age.

But there is yet another important factor that needs to be looked at: hunger.

Hunger seems to benefit your physical shape and longevity similarly to physical exercise. When manipulated properly, hunger has been shown to trigger mechanisms that increase your energy, repair your tissues, and keep you in a prime physical shape.

Let's take a closer look at hunger and how it affects your body.

Chapter 25

Hunger and Your Physical Shape

Hunger gives you the desire to eat. And incredibly, it also reflects your physical shape. It can make you lean and healthy, or it can make you fat and sick. That really depends on how your body is trained to endure lack of food and what kind of hunger you're experiencing.

There are two kinds of hunger: acute and chronic. And there is a huge difference in how they affect your body.

Acute hunger is a temporary sensation that is turned off by feeding. It's typically associated with a healthy metabolism and low body fat. Chronic hunger, on the other hand, is continuous and nonresponsive to feeding. That type of hunger has been linked to metabolic disorders and a tendency to gain weight.

To further understand how hunger works, we need to take a look at the physiological system behind it. Hunger is part of a powerful system that balances your energy intake and expenditure. Your hunger-satiety system consists of multiple neuropeptides that act to initiate or terminate your feeding.

These are your hunger and satiety hormones. Their signals are integrated by centers in your brain to modulate how you consume, spend, or store energy. And the balance between these signals dictates whether your body is in a fat-burning or a fat-storing mode.

In order to maintain a steady body weight, your hunger and satiety signals must continually adjust your food intake to your energy expenditure. Any imbalance between these two will affect your fat stores and physical shape.

Obesity, for instance, is an indication of a disrupted energy balance in which a surplus of accumulated energy is stored as body fat.

So what makes you lose control of your energy balance and physical shape? What can you do to regain these?

And how does all that relate to your hunger?

What Makes You Lose Control of Your Energy Balance and Physical Shape?

It has been argued that evolutionary pressure resulted in an overly strong human drive to eat when food is readily available. We evolved to thrive in a world where food wasn't easily accessible. Our original food was low-glycemic and fibrous—not the kind of food that typically promotes overeating. But we live today in a world of plenty, surrounded by foods that encourage consumption of excess energy.

So it is the disparity between the primordial environment of food scarcity in which we evolved to thrive and the current availability of excess food that contributes to unrestricted calorie consumption with the increasing prevalence of obesity and related diseases in our society.

But calorie consumption is only one factor. Emerging evidence indicates that there is another powerful factor behind the scene. And it's probably the most influential determinant of your energy status and physical shape.

You can be on a low-calorie diet and fail to lose weight, and you can be on a high-calorie diet and yet manage to slim down. That really depends on one factor: the balance between your hunger and satiety hormones.

How the Balance between Your Hunger and Satiety Hormones Affects Your Physical Shape

Your physical shape seems to depend on the ratio between your hunger and satiety hormones. Both hormones regulate your eating behavior, albeit with opposite effects on your body.

- Hunger hormones tend to slow your metabolism and make you gain weight.
- Satiety hormones act to boost your metabolism and help you slim down.

Your hunger and satiety hormones are consistently clashing with each other. They're divided into two groups that counteract each other's actions like two armies at war. And the consequences of that hormonal clash are manifested in your body.

Simply put, if your hunger hormones get out of control, you'll be prone to suffer from a declined metabolism and excess body fat. And if you let your satiety hormones take over, they will counteract the effects of your hunger hormones to allow you greater energy and a lean physique.

But that's merely a rough picture of your hunger-satiety system, and it doesn't yet fully explain how this system works.

The truth is that your hunger hormones aren't inherently bad. And when balanced, they play important roles in your metabolic system. Under healthy conditions they may even help you burn fat.

The hunger peptide ghrelin, for instance, is a most potent trigger of your growth hormone. Ghrelin binds to growth hormone secretagogue (GHS) receptors and increases its release by up to sixfold. Hence, fasting and hunger boost your growth hormone and potentiate its actions to burn fat and repair tissues.

Your hunger hormones are part of your survival apparatus. They relate to your satiety hormones like yin to yang. Hunger hormones give you the drive to search for food or hunt along with the desire to achieve. They keep you alert, and they balance the actions of your satiety hormones, which tend to calm you down. That's how your hunger hormones act under normal conditions.

But if your hunger-satiety system is disrupted and your hunger hormones get out of control, you may experience chronic hunger, diminished energy, metabolic decline, and an increased tendency to gain weight.

The point is that you need to know how to manipulate both types of hormones to work for you. And you certainly need to keep your hunger hormones under control. But before we address that, let's take an even closer look at your hunger and satiety hormones and how they affect your metabolism, body weight, and physical shape.

Your Hunger Hormones and Physical Shape

Your most notable hunger hormones are ghrelin, neuropeptide Y (NPY), and agouti-related protein (AgRP), all of which affect your body in the following ways:

- Decrease your energy expenditure
- Suppress your sympathetic nerve activity
- Inhibit your thyroid axis
- Reduce your body's thermogenesis (capacity to generate body heat)
- Inhibit your sex hormones
- Increase your stress hormone cortisol
- Increase your tendency to gain body fat

If left uncontrolled, hunger hormones will block the signals of your satiety hormones to reduce food intake, which may in turn lead to chronic cravings, uncontrollable food consumption, and excessive weight gain. And as you can see, they may also inhibit your primary sex hormones, suppress your libido, and spike your stress hormones.

What Makes Your Hunger Hormones Get Out of Control?

Normally, your hunger hormones are highly responsive to feeding. Their levels increase during fasting and reduce upon food ingestion.

During fasting, your hunger hormone ghrelin peaks while boosting your growth hormone to initiate fat burning and tissue repair. Meanwhile, your remaining hunger hormones are continuously counteracted and balanced by some of your satiety hormones (adiponectin and glucagon-like peptide), which are also responsive to fasting. This keeps your hunger under control and potentiates your sensitivity to satiety signals.

Then, when you resume eating, your hunger hormones decline, allowing your satiety hormones to kick in. And as your satiety hormones levels peak, they act to boost your metabolism.

That's how your hunger-satiety system is programmed to work under healthy conditions. It allows you to burn fat when you don't eat, and it boosts your metabolism when you eat.

Which is apparently a win-win situation.

But your hunger-satiety system can only function well as long as your diet is adequate. If your feeding episodes are too frequent and your foods are high-glycemic, your hunger-satiety system will be utterly disrupted.

Frequent incorporation of high-glycemic meals impairs your key satiety hormones insulin and leptin, leaving your hunger hormones unopposed and dominant. In case of insulin resistance, ghrelin levels remain elevated even after meal consumption—a condition that typically leads to chronic hunger (mostly for carbohydrates), excess food intake, and weight gain.

This issue has been widely overlooked, perhaps because people normally like to consume baking goods and candies on a daily basis and even more so during celebrations. Nonetheless, the evidence leaves no doubt: frequent consumption of high-glycemic foods jeopardizes your satiety system and puts your body under the tyranny of your hunger hormones.

To prevent that we need to take a look at your satiety hormones. How do they counteract your hunger hormones? And how do they affect your physical shape?

Your Satiety Hormones and Physical Shape

Your satiety hormones protect you against the effects of your hunger hormones. They act to sustain your energy and prevent metabolic decline. These include insulin, leptin, adiponectin, cholecystokinin (CCK), glucagon-like peptide (GLP), PPY, and melanocortins. When potentiated to dominate your hunger hormones, they affect your body in the following ways:

- Increase your energy expenditure
- Stimulate your thyroid axis
- Increase your sympathetic nerve activity
- Increase your body's thermogenesis
- Enhance your sex hormones
- Decrease your cortisol level
- Increase your capacity to burn fat

Your satiety hormones promote the right metabolic environment to allow you be at your leanest, healthiest, and most vigorous physical shape.

What Boosts Your Satiety Hormones?

Your satiety hormones are enhanced by three major factors:

- Food restriction
- Exercise
- Weight loss

Food restriction, exercise, and weight loss significantly increase the sensitivity and effectiveness of your insulin and leptin, and they potentiate the actions of your melanocortin and adiponectin.

This indicates that with proper diet, exercise, and restoration of a healthy body weight, you can increase the efficiency of your satiety hormones to allow you to achieve peak physical potential.

Soon we'll see how all this translates into practice, but for now let's continue with your most potent satiety hormones, insulin and leptin, which are pivotal to keeping your metabolism intact.

How Insulin and Leptin Affect Your Metabolism

Insulin is your most important satiety hormone. It regulates your sex hormones, muscle buildup, blood sugar, and energy levels. Insulin sensitivity is essential to keeping your testosterone and libido intact.

And insulin resistance leads to testosterone decline and loss of sex drive.

Insulin sensitivity is also necessary for normal leptin activity.

Leptin is one of your most powerful metabolic-boosting hormones. Secreted from your adipose tissue, it's a peptide hormone that primarily lowers your food intake, boosts your metabolic rate, increases your energy expenditure, and decreases your body fat. It enhances your thyroid activity and contributes to the sustainability of your immune system. Absence of leptin has been shown to cause a severe metabolic decline and morbid obesity.

But again, leptin can't act without insulin. Both hormones share a common signaling pathway, and they get impaired (resistant) by the same causes.

What Causes Insulin and Leptin Resistance?

The main cause of insulin and leptin resistance is excess body fat and particularly visceral fat, which is the adipose tissue that surrounds the inner organs. The most trivial dietary cause is food that combines high sugar with high fat.

It has been found that the high sugar–high fat combo causes insulin and leptin resistance even prior to any change in body composition. This means that all food products made with a high content of sugar and fat—including cookies, cakes, ice creams, and chocolates—are poisonous to your satiety system. And they set you up for serious metabolic disorders associated with insulin and leptin resistance, which may include excess circulating estrogen, excess cortisol, declining testosterone, blood sugar disorders, and a tendency to gain stubborn belly fat.

The good news is that both insulin and leptin resistance could be reversed by food restriction and weight loss.

Hence, both hormones are enhanced by austerity and shattered by indulgence. It has therefore been suggested that insulin and leptin play important roles in times of scarcity but have a lesser role in times of plenty.

How Do You Put Your Satiety Hormones in Charge of Your Body?

There are two ways to literally achieve that:

1. Train your body to endure hunger.
2. Eat foods that promote satiety.

Train Your Body to Endure Hunger

Hunger should be treated like physical exercise. Both hunger and exercise are perceived by your body as survival signals to adapt and improve.

When your body is methodically challenged with acute hunger, it adjusts itself accordingly. Incredibly, periodical fasting and acute hunger cause a decrease in your brain's hunger receptors, which makes you even more capable of resisting hunger. This in turn enables your satiety hormones to get increasingly efficient, allowing them to overpower your hunger hormones and take control of your metabolism.

But only real hunger can benefit you that way. Real hunger is what you experience while fasting or undereating, not the kind of cravings you feel on a full belly.

There are a few ways to train your body to endure hunger. You can try to gradually increase the gap between your meals or alternatively put your body in an undereating state for most of the day. And you can also try exercising while fasting.

Let's see how all this translates into practice.

Undereating

You can put your body in an undereating state by minimizing your food intake during the day to small, low-glycemic protein meals every three to four hours. These could be served with (or substituted with) green vegetables or small servings of low-glycemic fruits such as berries, green apples, or pomegranates.

Undereating has some notable advantages. It challenges your body similar to fasting, yielding a negative energy balance that promotes fat burning and tissue recycling. But unlike fasting, it allows you to nourish your muscle with protein and antioxidants, and you won't feel the desire to eat as intensely as when you completely avoid food.

But whether you fast or undereat, do not chronically restrict your calories.

Your hunger must be acute, not chronic. Treat yourself with sufficient food in your main meal to compensate for the energy and nutrients you spend during the day.

Exercising While Fasting

Probably the most intense way to improve your hunger durability is by exercising while fasting. This presents a double challenge to your body, and it yields a stronger impact than fasting or exercise alone.

Though training while fasting may initially affect your maximum performance, it will nevertheless come with an additional bonus.

A study published in the *Journal of Physiology* in November 2010 indicated that exercising while fasting increases the body's metabolic adaptation efficiency to utilize energy, burn fat, and deposit protein in the muscle, and substantially more so than when exercising after a meal.

The researchers reported that the increased capacity to deposit protein in the muscle as observed in people who were exercising while fasting and then eating a postexercise meal is a result of increased insulin sensitivity and activation of the muscle mTOR (the mechanism that builds muscle).

Your body is inherently programmed to benefit from enduring hunger via fasting, undereating, and exercising while fasting. But that durability can be even further enhanced by satiety-promoting foods.

Foods That Promote Satiety

The food that promotes satiety most is protein. It has been reported that protein promotes satiety more effectively than carbohydrates or fat. Out of all proteins, the one with the fastest satiety impact is whey protein. Studies reveal that consumption of whey protein before meals can swiftly boost the satiety peptides CCK and GLP-1, which have been shown to decrease food intake and increase weight loss.

Whey protein is also beneficial when consumed before exercise. Having a small serving of whey protein (with no added sugar) about thirty minutes before exercise seems to yield the same benefits as exercising while fasting. And it comes with an additional bonus: a pre-exercise whey meal can help you sustain intense performance, which could be compromised if you train while fasting.

Other satiety-promoting foods are raw nuts, seeds, legumes, roots, and greens. Being low-glycemic and fibrous, these plant foods are a great fit for your insulin/leptin system. Nuts and seeds trigger a satiety peptide called PPY, which is highly sensitive to dietary fat.

PPY increases your metabolic efficiency and shifts your cravings from carbohydrates to fat. That action is contrary to your hunger hormones, which generally shift your cravings toward carbohydrates.

Note that it's the shift toward refined carbohydrates that has been linked to excessive food intake. Refined carbohydrates overspike your insulin and disrupt your satiety apparatus. This is the reason why once you start eating potato chips, you may find it difficult to stop.

But again, nothing is more damaging to your satiety than the combination of high sugar and high fat. This dietary combo packs on calories, damages your insulin, and shatters your satiety along with your whole metabolic system.

Finally, realize that time is a factor. The longer you train your body to endure hunger and enjoy the subtle taste of satiety foods such as quality whole protein, nuts, seeds, roots, legumes, fresh greens, and low-glycemic fruits, the more adapted and sensitive to satiety you'll get.

And note that your muscle literally thrives on satiety foods. Combinations of foods such as whey and berries, eggs and beans, or meat and nuts have unmatched muscle-nourishing properties. Furthermore, being satiety oriented, these food combinations promote the right hormonal environment for muscle conditioning and buildup.

Summary and Projections

Understanding the biological system that regulates hunger and satiety along with energy balance is a key to preventing eating disorders, metabolic decline, muscle waste, and undesirable weight gain.

More studies are needed to elucidate the relationship between human nutrition and survival. As the mechanisms of feeding and energy homeostasis are studies and clarified, treatments based on the natural manipulation of hunger and satiety could be just as effective as hormonal therapy in adjusting hormonal disorders and deficiency.

Manipulations of hunger and satiety may be useful in restoring thyroid hormone activity, balancing estrogen, and attenuating or even preventing the age-related decline of growth hormone and testosterone.

These strategies may help affect the enormous morbidity associated with obesity and related diseases. And they may also help eliminate the life-threatening risks associated with hormone replacement therapies and chemical drugs.

In today's world you need to know what your best options are. In this case, nature doesn't leave you with many choices. Controlling hunger is not an option; it's a necessity.

Chapter 26

Conclusion

Evolutionary biology and physical anthropology provide us with substantial data to figure out which foods and exercises fit our biological needs most. Today we can identify the core principles upon which our diet and training should be based.

The Human Diet's Three Overruling Principles

Biologists continue to recognize distinct evolutionary features of human food selection and eating behavior that indicate adaptation to a specific diet. And based on the enormous information available to us, we can conclude that our original diet is based on three principles:

1. It's exclusively whole food oriented.
2. It's primarily low-glycemic.
3. It's inherently more vegetarian than carnivorous.

Note that these principles apply to all humans and overrule the differences between body types and genetic predispositions.

Here are the facts:

- **We're programmed for whole-food nutrition.** Our bodies have not evolved to accept anything synthetic or refined without suffering side effects. Synthetic substances include all drugs, artificial food additives, synthetic vitamins, and industrial chemicals.

Refined foods include all protein isolates, simple and refined carbohydrates, and refined oils.

- **We're programmed for a low-glycemic diet.** The low-glycemic diet benefits our hormonal and muscular systems. It's inherently satiety-oriented and has been shown to promote a healthy metabolism, lean physique, and longevity.

Conversely, high-glycemic diets have been shown to shatter insulin and lead to obesity, diabetes, cardiovascular disease, and a shorter life span.

- **Plant foods are essential to us. Animal foods are not.** Vegetables, fruits, nuts, seeds, legumes, and roots are our primary sources of vitamins and antioxidants. They're also exclusive sources of metabolic-supportive phytonutrients.

  Proper combinations of vegetables, seeds, nuts and legumes can yield a complete protein and provide us with all the essential nutrients we need. And even though plant foods yield protein with a lower bioavailability than that of animal foods, they nonetheless provide us with the essential nutrient complexity required to sustain life, which is missing in animal food.

  This means that we can live on plant food alone, but we can't depend on animal food as our sole source of nutrients.

- **We're originally programmed to consume seeds and nuts as our main staple foods.** Human jaw and teeth morphology bear proof to this. Seeds and nuts are satiety-oriented and insulin-friendly. They provide us with protein, fiber, essential oil, fat-soluble vitamins, antioxidants, metabolic-supportive phytonutrients, and low-glycemic fuel needed to keep our metabolic system intact.

- **We're programmed for a diet of primarily solid food.** We digest better when we chew solid food and predigest it with our saliva. Our cheek teeth are originally structured for chewing solid food with a crunch. And the food's texture seems to contribute to our satiety.

Liquid diets lack that solid texture and therefore may fail to yield complete satiety. Hence, liquid diets may lead to chronic cravings, excess food intake, and related adverse effects.

That said, quality whey protein shakes can be highly beneficial as functional muscle meals due to their fast nutrient delivery, but by themselves they aren't sufficient to constitute a complete diet.

The Human Feeding Cycle

Our feeding is regulated by the autonomic nervous system, which controls how we select food, how much we eat, and how often.

Our autonomic nervous system is geared toward nocturnal eating. It rejects feeding during the stressful hours of the day and encourages eating during the calming hours of the night.

Scientists believe that this feeding cycle originated in primordial times of food scarcity, which forced humans to endure physical hardship while fasting for most of the day. And since early humans were primarily day hunters (as manifested in our poor night vision), it only makes sense that our original rest and feeding time would be at night.

Night is the biologically right time for having our largest meal of the day.

Shifting between A.M. Food and P.M. Food

The human feeding cycle is positively correlated with our wake/sleep cycle. Its premise is to gradually shift from A.M. to P.M. foods. A.M. foods are primarily light and raw, whereas P.M. foods are denser and cooked.

This dietary shift serves a clear biological purpose. It accommodates the changes in our hormonal system and metabolic needs throughout the day and night. During the day, it lets us spend energy, remove toxins, burn fat, and stay alert. And during the night, it enables us to replenish nutrients, recuperate, relax, and sleep.

The human feeding cycle is essential for all the key mechanisms that make us thrive:

- It keeps our insulin sensitive.
- It keeps our satiety system in charge.
- It keeps our hormonal/metabolic system intact.

The rotation between A.M. and P.M. feeding is critical for the viability of our diet. Yet it's still ignored and denied by mainstream nutrition.

Mainstream nutrition authorities gave us the wrong food pyramid and the wrong diets. And they failed to provide us with solid criteria upon which we can judge whether we eat right or wrong. Most of us have no clue what the human feeding cycle even means.

But we can't ignore the facts, and we can't dismiss what we already know: virtually all current diets have been failing miserably.

Our society has been getting consistently fatter and sicker even though we're dieting more than ever. And unless we adjust our feeding cycle to accommodate our biological needs, we'll continue paying the consequences with our health and physical shape.

Human Training

Humans are inherently programmed for a specific kind of training. The regimen that has demonstrated the most proven record in maximizing human performance is the short intense training protocol. This regimen yields the most impressive results in building muscle and preventing its degradation and aging.

But the intensity and duration of training are not the only determinates of human physical conditioning. We still need to know what kind of exercises we are originally programmed for.

What Kind of Exercises Are We Originally Programmed For?

Like other animals, we evolved to benefit from physical activities that were essential to the survival of our species. Being a predator species, our survival depended largely on our hunting activities. Based on skeleton and joint morphology, we exhibit features of pack hunters and ambush predators combined. And we behave accordingly.

We tend to gather in groups like pack hunters or act alone like ambush predators. These predatory features are inherent to us, and they dictate how we're programmed to behave even if we aren't aware of that. The point is: our predatory nature must be recognized as a key factor in designing our physical conditioning.

That's the way we're programmed to act, and that's how we're destined to train.

Wolf People versus Cat People

The idea that we originated as a killer species may seem extreme to most people. Needless to say how controversial it may be to ask people to adjust their training to accommodate their primitive predatory nature.

That idea might sound far-fetched. But it makes more biological sense than all other fitness theories. Not only does it make sense, it actually enables us to establish authentic criteria of human training. And it finally takes out the "vague factor." Human training is not a random collection of exercises. And it certainly isn't about running on a treadmill to nowhere. Human fitness has a biological purpose.

We can now understand what that purpose is.

Biological fitness means physical adaptation for better survival. Our survival depends on adaptability to hardship. Each of us carries an innate survival program with a defined fight-or-flight mechanism that enables us to adapt and improve to better survive. We need to practice that survival program. And we certainly need to integrate it in our training routines.

That's the only way to unlock the mechanisms that transform our bodies from normal to supreme shape, enabling us to achieve our true biological potential.

So what kind of activities are we inherently programmed for?

Humans are divided in their affinities to sport activities. Some people like team sports, whereas others prefer individual sports. Some prefer wolflike activities that involve pursuit and chasing such as soccer, whereas others prefer catlike activities such as grappling, wrestling, or boxing. And some prefer power drills, which seem to complement both types of activities.

It's quite funny to notice how a wolf person and a cat person behave in times of adversity, such as when confronting a foe. A wolf person will stick his face in front of his rival's face as if ready to bite, whereas a cat person will keep a distance, ready to strike with his hands.

Wolf people seem to prefer leg drills (running), whereas cat people seem to prefer hand drills (punching, grappling, or weight lifting). Nonetheless, each of us is programmed for both types of activities. So despite the differences between our personal training affinities, we need to exercise both options.

But whether you're primarily a wolf or a cat person, you should be aware of one important physical trait that is inherent to our species yet is often overlooked or denied. It's called the aggressive hand concept.

The Aggressive Hand Concept

According to biologists Raymond Dart and Clark Howell, humans evolved to routinely use their hands not just for daily chores, but also for intimidating social rivals or fighting an enemy. Hence, strong hands were a social and survival necessity. Having the capacity for hand-to-hand combat was apparently a primal human trait. Darwin called that "the aggressive hand concept."

The aggressive hand concept reflects how we're programmed to use our hands when facing a physical threat. Other apes tend to use their teeth more than their forearms for intimidating and fighting (biting).

It seems that behind our civilized appearance there's a "handy" predator waiting to strike.

The aggressive hand concept is almost exclusively human. Unlike other species, we use our hands in virtually every physical and cognitive task. This includes toiling, striking, grappling, writing, playing music, and even speaking. We use our hands to dictate our legs' speed when we sprint, and we use them to maximize our force output when we jump.

Our hand and arm muscles are substantially more innervated in our brains than our leg muscles are. We literally think with our hands. And we're the only species capable of doing that.

The benefit of keeping our hand-shoulder complex strong and viable may go beyond the physical. We need capable hands to accommodate both our physical and mental capacities.

Hunger and Satiety

Our physical shape is largely controlled by hunger and satiety hormones. The balance between these hormones dictates whether we tend to be lean and healthy or overweight and sick. Hunger hormones generally tend to slow our metabolism and make us gain weight, whereas satiety hormones tend to boost our metabolism and make us slim down.

Under normal conditions these hormones balance each other to allow optimum energy and a healthy metabolism. But most people today have lost that balance. Most people are chronically hungry, overfed, and overweight.

We have been shifting away from our primal satiety-oriented diet, and we certainly suffer the consequences.

The Shift from Satiety to Hunger

The shift from satiety to hunger has to do with the disparity between the world in which we originally evolved to thrive and the world in which we live today. We evolved to thrive in a world of scarcity, nourished by foods that promoted satiety, but we live today in a world of plenty, surrounded by foods that promote hunger. And instead of being lean, strong, and muscular, most of us today are overweight, weak, and soft.

The shift from satiety to hunger is even more damaging.

The vast majority of people today are prone to suffer from premature aging. This has to do with the loss of two primary satiety-oriented hormones: insulin and testosterone.

We're a testosterone-driven species. Pound for pound, humans have more testosterone than any other species on this planet. But testosterone is insulin-dependent, and insulin is our major satiety hormone. Since we've been shifting away from satiety foods and shattering our insulin, we've been consistently losing our testosterone. It has been estimated that the average modern man has been losing 1 percent of his testosterone every year.

In addition to that, we have been losing our growth hormone.

We're originally programmed to boost our growth hormone when fasting throughout the day. But most people today can't endure hunger, so they eat too frequently while chronically inhibiting their growth hormone. Consequently, as people get older, they experience symptoms of premature aging, which include waste of muscle and bone tissues, loss of strength, and a persistent metabolic decline.

Most people today are food addicts. The typical diet is based on high-glycemic foods that act like addictive substances, keeping people hungry and craving for more. Hunger-promoting foods shatter insulin, diminish testosterone, and suppress growth hormone.

And if that's not bad enough, people today are commonly exposed to hunger-inducing substances, which are abundantly found in processed food products. These include MSG (as typically found in food flavoring, hydrolyzed yeast, hydrolyzed proteins, and hydrolyzed grains), industrial fructose, artificial sweeteners, and sugar alcohol. These substances shatter satiety by disrupting insulin and binding to brain opioid receptors (addiction receptors), which stimulate hunger and suppress satiety.

The Solution

The solution must be drastic. Our society's state of health has been manipulated by hunger-promoting foods and substances. We need to train ourselves to shift back into a satiety-oriented diet. We must eat right and eat less frequently!

This obviously goes against industrial interests.

If we give up all refined flours, simple sugars, fructose, MSG, synthetic additives, sugar alcohol, and artificial sweeteners, we will devastate the current food industry and literally shut down most sport nutrition and supplement companies.

But as drastic as this solution may seem, it's the only way to overcome our health crisis. There is no way around it. Biologically, we're programmed for a satiety-oriented, whole-food diet. Our hormonal and muscular systems are satiety-oriented, and so is our health.

We need to change our diet approach. No more "cheat days," and no more "everything is allowed in moderation . . ."

Nothing but 100-percent natural, low-glycemic, whole food can make us thrive.

Supplementation

Since the typical diet isn't always sufficient to cover the minimum requirements for essential and antioxidant nutrients, there is a reasonable need to use nutritional supplements. Supplementation allows you to nourish your body with high concentrations of essential food nutrients and thereby support your metabolic needs along with your hormonal, neural, and muscular systems.

But only food-based supplements can do this job.

Synthetic supplements should be avoided. These have been shown to disrupt muscle energy production and impair adaptability to exercise. Synthetic vitamins and antioxidants may be useful in clinical cases, such as immunodeficiencies or digestive insufficiencies, but they should always be treated cautiously like drugs.

You should also avoid yeast-based supplements. Yeast is a major allergen; it's a bacterial product that contains MSG and may cause severe reactions along with neurotoxicity, which altogether present a serious health concern.

Unlock Your Muscle Genes

Your muscle genes are highly responsive to nutritional and physical triggers. They're activated by hardship and suppressed by indulgence.

Your muscle machinery is programmed for generating supreme power, and it's constantly humming ready for action. But your muscular system is shackled by an innate inhibitory mechanism that puts the brakes on your muscle strength and development, prohibiting it from reaching its peak power potential.

To counteract your muscle inhibition, you need to use the right physical and nutritional triggers. When your muscle genes are triggered, a cascade of cellular events takes place, allowing your muscle to recycle broken proteins and damaged cells, upgrade fiber quality, maximize force production, and resist aging.

Your Muscle Genes' Triggers

The main triggers of your muscle genes are

1. Insulin
2. Exercise/mechanical overload
3. Amino acids
4. Fasting

Insulin

Insulin is your primary muscle trigger. The insulin pathway is your muscle's main support system. It's essential for turning on your muscle genes; it controls your muscle mTOR; and it potentiates your most powerful muscle-building hormones—testosterone, growth hormone, and insulin-like growth factors. Any impairment in your insulin will disrupt all anabolic processes and lead to muscle degradation and wasting.

Exercise/Mechanical Overload

Mechanical overload is the key physical trigger of your muscle mTOR. The overload impact from intense weight lifting and explosive drills drives mTOR to increase protein synthesis in your muscle toward repair and growth.

Mechanical overload is the trigger that turns on your myosin heavy chain (MHC) genes to develop your fast muscle fibers. It also triggers myogenic regulatory factors (MRFs) to convert satellite cells into myoblasts, which then fuse into new muscle cells. This process upgrades your muscle fiber quality and keeps your muscle young, strong, and durable.

Amino Acids

The main nutritional triggers of your muscle are amino acids, particularly leucine. Leucine directly turns on your muscle mTOR; its impact is almost as potent as an anabolic steroid. But in order to grant a real anabolic effect, your leucine intake must be high (over 8 g per day).

Leucine is part of the branched-chain amino acids (BCAAs). The BCAAs isoleucine and valine spare leucine from wasting as energy substrate and shift it instead to its anabolic pathway. The higher your intake of BCAA is, the more anabolic your meal is. But only dietary BCAA can fully benefit your muscle without side effects (intravenous administration of free-form BCAA has been shown to cause severe insulin resistance).

This means that the most effective muscle meals are those made with protein foods rich in BCAA. The best food sources of BCAA and leucine are dairy proteins, out of which whey protein comes on top.

Fasting

Fasting affects your muscle similar to physical exercise. Besides stabilizing your insulin and accelerating fat burning, fasting activates genes and growth factors that regenerate new brain and muscle cells.

In the brain, fasting turns on brain-derived neurotrophic factor (BDNF), which activates stem cells, making them committed to restore and regenerate new neurons. In the muscle, BDNF acts to protect neuromotors from degradation while activating satellite cells to commit, differentiate, and fuse into new muscle cells.

Fasting is the most powerful trigger of muscle tissue recycling. It increases the removal of broken proteins and damaged cells to allow the synthesis of new protein and regeneration of new muscle cells for repair and rejuvenation. It also boosts growth hormone by six- to tenfold and thereby yields a substantial anti-aging effect on the bone and muscle tissues.

Given this, periodical (intermittent) fasting may prove to be a most effective anti-aging strategy—and even more so when combined with exercise.

Muscle Rejuvenation versus Muscle Buildup

You need to define your main fitness goal. Is it muscle rejuvenation or muscle buildup? Muscle rejuvenation and muscle buildup are not the same. They require different strategies. And even though these two seem to go hand in hand, the first is about tissue recycling and keeping your muscles young, whereas the second is more about protein deposit toward muscle gain. Let's review the differences:

Muscle Rejuvenation

For muscle rejuvenation, you need to initiate muscle catabolism for the removal and recycling of broken proteins and damaged cells. And along with this, you need to turn on the mechanism that signals satellite cells in your muscle to commit and convert into new muscle cells.

The best way to do this is by combining intermittent fasting with short intense exercise. Exercising while fasting seems to be the most effective way to maximize the recycling and rejuvenation effects on your muscle tissues.

As a general rule, have one to two recovery meals made with fast-assimilating proteins (whey protein) right after your workout. Feeding your muscle after exercise with fast-assimilating proteins is needed to stop the catabolic process in your muscle and shift the recycling process toward repair and growth.

Remember, both parts of this regimen are critically important—both the catabolic (fasting/exercise) and anabolic (feeding) components are essential to the rejuvenation of your muscle.

Muscle Buildup

For muscle buildup, you need to promote muscle anabolism and inhibit muscle breakdown. It has been commonly believed that muscle buildup requires a daily intake of 1 to 2 g protein per pound of body weight. This means an extremely high daily intake of protein—about 2 to 4 pounds of meat, chicken, or fish or fifty eggs per day for a 170-pound person.

But there is another way to achieve that, apparently a more efficient one. Called pulse feeding, it involves a frequent use of small, fast-assimilating, low-glycemic whey protein meals (with no sugar added) throughout the day, including two to three postexercise recovery meals.

Pulse-feeding of this type has a proven record of success. It has been shown to yield maximum protein utilization efficiency in the muscle with minimum digestive stress and without overspiking insulin. Here is how it technically works.

The incorporation of small whey protein meals throughout the day grants complete protein utilization from each meal. Twenty grams net protein is the threshold needed to yield max utilization efficiency. So when combining six whey meals (20 g net protein each), you get a minimum 100 to 120 g net protein utilized in your body before even starting your evening meal.

Let's put the record straight regarding protein utilization. The typical protein utilization efficiency from "normal" meals is less than 40 percent. Hence, you normally waste at least 60 percent of the protein you get from your diet. So to get 100 g net protein utilization, you need to consume 250 g protein, which you get from about 2.5 pounds of meat or 40 eggs per day . . . lots of protein and digestive stress to handle.

In comparison, pulse feeding with frequent, small whey meals allows you to get the same anabolic effect from a much lower net protein intake (less than third) and with minimum digestive stress or side effects.

Body Transformation

It may take some time to adjust your training and eating routines, and it may take even longer to transform your body. But it doesn't take long to trigger your muscle genes. And as long as you keep your muscle genes unlocked, every minute will count in resetting your body's biological clock backward and get you closer to achieving your peak physical potential.

Final Note

Getting biologically fit in today's world is not an easy goal. You need courage to go against the trend and a great determination to fight the elements. And you need a relentless desire to succeed. If you have the heart for this, I believe you'll acquire a sense of power you may have never experienced before. Remember, your body thrives when challenged; it turns pain to power. Take advantage of that—enjoy this power.

References

Acheson, A., J. C. Conover, J. P. Fandl, T. M. DeChiara, M. Russell, A. Thadani, S. P. Squinto, G. D. Yancopoulos, and R. M. Lindsay. "A BDNF Autocrine Loop in Adult Sensory Neurons Prevents Cell Death." *Nature* 374, no. 6521 (1995): 450–53.

Ahima, R. S., D. Prabakaran, C. Mantzoros, D. Qu, B. Lowell, E. Maratos-Flier, and J. S. Flier. "Role of Leptin in the Neuroendrocine Response to Fasting." *Nature* 382 (1996): 250–52.

Air, E. L., M. Z. Strowski, S. C. Benoit, S. L. Conarello, G. M. Salituro, X. M. Guan, K. Liu, S. C. Woods, and B. B. Zhang. "Small Molecule Insulin Mimetics Reduce Food Intake and Body Weight and Prevent Development of Obesity." *Nature Medicine* 8 (2002): 179–83.

Andersson, U., K. Filipsson, C. R. Abbott, A. Woods, K. Smiht, S. R. Bloom, D. Carling, and C. J. Small. "AMP-Activated Protein Kinase Plays a Role in the Control of Food Intake." *Journal of Biological Chemistry* 279 (2004): 12005–8.

Araujo, A. B., V. Kupelian, S. T. Page, D. J. Handelsman, W. K. Bremner, and J. B. McKinlay. "Sex Steroids and All-Cause and Cause-Specific Mortality in Men." *Arch Intern Med* 167, no. 12 (2007): 1252–60.

Argyropoulos, G., T. Rankinen, D. R. Neufeld, T. Rice, M. A. Province, A. S. Leon, J. S. Skinner, J. H. Wilmore, D. C. Rao, and C. Bouchard. "A Polymorphism in the Human Agouti-Related Protein Is Associated with Late-Onset Obesity." *Journal of Clinical Endocrinology and Metabolism* 87 (2002): 4198–202.

Arita, Y., S. Kihara, N. Ouchi, M. Takahaski, K. Maeda, J. Miyagawa, K. Hotta, I. Shimomura, T. Nakamura, K. Miyaoka, et al. "Paradoxical Decrease of an Adipose-Specific Protein, Adiponectin, in Obesity." *Biochemical and Biophysical Research Communications* 257 (1999): 79–83.

Arnal, M. A., L. Mosoni, Y. Boirie, M. L. Houlier, L. Morin, E. Verdier, P. Ritz, J. M. Antoine, J. Prugnaud, B. Beaufrere, et al. "Protein Pulse

Feeding Improves Protein Retention in Elderly Women." *Am. J. Clinical Nutrition* 69, no. 6 (1999): 1202–8.

Aziz, E., E. L. Brainerd, and T. J. Roberts. "Variable Gearing in Pennate Muscles." *Proceedings the National Academy of Sciences of the USA* 105 (2008): 1745–50.

Bagnasco, M., M. G. Dube, P. S. Kalra, and S. P. Kalra. "Evidence for the Existence of Distinct Central Appetite, Energy Expenditure, and Ghrelin Stimulation Pathways as Revealed by Hypothalamic Site-Specific Leptin Gene Therapy." *Endocrinology* 143 (2002): 4409–21.

Balthasar, N., R. Coppari, J. McMinn, S. M. Liu, C. E. Lee, V. Tang, C. D. Kenny, R. A. McGovern, S. C. Chua Jr., J. K. Elmquist, and B. B. Lowell. "Leptin Receptor of Signaling in POMC Neurons Is Required for Normal Body Weight Homeostasis." *Neuron* 42 (2004): 983–91.

Banks, W. A. "The source of Cerebral Insulin." *European Journal of Pharmacology* 490 (2004): 5–12.

Banks, W. A., C. R. DiPalma, and C. L. Farrell. "Impaired Transport of Leptin across the Blood-Brain Barrier in Obesity." *Peptides* 20 (1999): 1341–45.

Banks, W. A., A. J. Kastin, W. Huang, J. B. Jaspan, and L. M. Maness. "Leptin Enters the Brain by a Saturable System Independent of Insulin." *Peptides* 17 (1996): 305–11.

Bath, K. G., and F. S. Lee. "Variant BDNF (Val66Met) Impact on Brain Structure and Function." *Cogn. Affect. Behav. Neurosci.* 6, no. 1 (2006): 79–85.

Baum, J. I., D. K. Layman, G. G. Freund, K. A. Rahn, M. T. Nakamura, and B. E. Yudell. "A Reduced Carbohydrate, Increased Protein Diet Stabilizes Glycemic Control and Minimizes Adipose Tissue Glucose Disposal in Rats." *J. Nutr.* 136, no. 7 (2006): 1855–61.

Baum, J. I., J. E. Seyler, J. C. O'Conner, G. G. Freund, and D. K. Layman. "The Effect of Leucine on Glucose Homeostasis and the Insulin Signaling Pathway. *FASEB J.* 17 (2003): A811.

Bauman, J. "The Strength of the Chimpanzee and the Orang." *Scientific Monthly* 16 (1923): 432–39.

Beglinger, C., L. Degen, D. Matzinger, M. D'Amato, and J. Drewe. "Loxiglumide, a CCK-A Receptor Antagonist, Stimulates Calorie Intake and Hunger Feelings in Humans." *American Journal of Physiology Regulatory, Integrative and Comparative Physiology* 280 (2001): R1149–54.

Bekinschtein, P., M. Cammarola, C. Katche, L. Slipczuk, J. I. Rossato, A. Goldin, I. Izquierdo, and J. H. Medina. "BDNF Is Essential to Promote Persistence of Long-Term Memory Storage." *Proc. Natl. Acad. Sci. U.S.A.* 105, no. 7 (2008): 2711–6.

Bernardis, L. I., and L. L. Bellinger. "The Lateral Hypothalamic Area Revisited: Ingestive Behavior." *Neuroscience and Biobehavioral Reviews* 20 (1996): 189–287.

Berridge, K. C. "Modulation of Taste Affect by Hunger, Calorie Satiety, and Sensory-Specific Satiety in the Rat." *Appetite* 16 (1991): 103–20.

Binder, D. K., and H. E. Scharfman. "Brain-Derived Neurotrophic Factor." *Growth Factors* 22, no. 3 (2004): 123–31.

Boirie, Y., M. Dangin, P. Gachon, M.-P. Vasson, J.-L. Maubois, and B. Beaufrere. "Slow and Fast Dietary Proteins Differently Modulate Postprandial Protein Accretion." Laboratoire de Nutrition Humaine, University Clermont Auvergne, Centre de Recherche en Nutrition Humaine, BP 321 (1997): 6.

Bottinelli, R. "Functional Heterogeneity of Mammalian Single Muscle Fibres: Do Myosin Isoforms Tell the Whole Story?" *Pflugers Archiv. Euro. Jour. of Physiology* 443 (2001): 6–17.

Boutrif, E. "Recent Developments in Protein Quality Evaluation." *Food, Nutrition and Agriculture* 2, no. 3 (1991): 36–40.

Bramble, D. M., and D. E. Lieberman. "Endurance Running and the Evolution of Homo." *Nature* 432 (2004): 345–352.

Bronstein, D. M., M. K. Schafer, S. J. Watson, and H. Akil. "Evidence That Beta-Endorphin Is Synthesized in Cells in the Nucleus Tractus Solitaries: Detection of POMC mRNA." *Brain Research* 584 (1992): 269–75.

Bruning, J. C., D. Gautam, D. J. Burks, J. Gillette, M. Schubert, P. C. Orban, R. Klein, W. Krone, D. Meiler-Wieland, and C. R. Kahn. "Role of Brain Insulin Receptor in Control of Body Weight and Reproduction." *Science* 289 (2000): 2122–25.

Brunoni, R., M. Lopes, and F. Fregni. "A Systematic Review and Meta-Analysis of Clinical Studies on Major Depression and BDNF Levels: Implications for the Role of Neuroplasticity in Depression." *International Journal of Neuropsychopharmacology* 11, no. 8 (2008): 1169.

Burks, D. J., J. F. de Mora, M. Schubert, D. J. Withers, M. G. Myers, H. H. Towery, S. L. Altamuro, C. L. Flint, and M. F. White. "IRS-2 Pathways Integrate Female Reproduction and Energy Homeostasis." *Nature* 407 (2000): 377–82.

Chan, J. L., K. Heist, A. M. DePaoli, J. D. Veldhuis, and C. S. Mantzoros. "The Role of Falling Leptin Levels in the Neuroendocrine and Metabolic Adaptation to Short-Term Starvation in Healthy Men." *Journal of Clinical Investigation* 111 (2003): 1409–1421.

Charge, S. B., and M. A. Rudnicki. "Cellular and Molecular Regulation of Muscle Regeneration." *Physiol Rev* 84 (2004): 209–38.

Chen, H., O. Charlat, L. A. Tartaglia, E. A. Woolf, X. Weng, S. J. Ellis, N. D. Lakey, J. Culpepper, K. J. Moore, R. E. Breitbart, G. M. Duyk, R. I. Tepper, and J. P. Morgenstern. "Evidence That the Diabetes Gene Encodes the Leptin Receptor: Identification of a Mutation in the Leptin Receptor Gene in db/db Mice." *Cell* 84 (1996): 491–45.

Cheung, C. C., D. K. Clifton, and R. A. Steiner. "Proopiomelanocortin Neurons Are Direct Targets for Leptin in the Hypothalamus." *Endocrinology* 138 (1997): 4489–92.

Chevrel, G., R. Hohlfeld, and M. Sendtner. "The Role of Neurotrophins in Muscle under Physiological and Pathopsychological Conditions." *Muscle Nerve* 33 (2006): 462–76.

Clow, C., and B. J. Jasmin. "Brain-Derived Neurotrophic Factor Regulates Satellite Cell Differentiation and Skeletal Muscle Regeneration." *Cell Physiology* 21, no. 13 (2010): 2182–90.

Cope, T. C., and M. J. Pinter. "The Size Principle: Still Working after All These Years." *News in Physiological Sciences* 10 (1995): 280–86.

Cotman, C. W., and N. C. Berchtold. "Exercise: A Behavioral Intervention to Enhance Brain Health and Plasticity." *Trends Neurosci.* 25, no. 6 (2002): 295–301.

Crawley, J. N., and R. L. Corwin. "Biological Actions of Cholecystokinin." *Peptides* 15 (1994): 731–55.

Cummings, D. E., R. S. Frayo, C. Marmonier, R. Aubert, and D. Chapelot. "Plasma Ghrelin Levels and Hunger Scores among Humans Initiating Meals Voluntarily in the Absence of Time- and Food-Related Cues." *American Journal of Physiology—Endocrinology and Metabolism* 287 (2004): E297–304.

Cummings, D. E., J. Q. Purnell, R. S. Frayo, K. Schmidova, B. E. Wisse, and D. S. Weigle. "A Preprandial Rise in Plasma Ghrelin Levels Suggests a Role in Meal Initiation in Humans." *Diabetes* 50 (2001): 1714–19.

Dart, R. A. "The Predatory Implemental Technique of *Australopithecus.*" *Am. J. Phys. Anthrop.* 7 (1949): 1–38.

Date, Y., M. Kojima, H. Hosoda, A. Sawaguchi, M. S. Mondal, T. Sugamuma, S. Marsukura, K. Kangawa, and M. Nakazato. "Ghrelin, a Novel Growth Hormone-Releasing Acylated Peptide, Is Synthesized in a Distinct Endocrine Cell Type in the Gastrointestinal Tracts of Rats and Humans." *Endocrinology* 141 (2000): 4255–61.

Date, Y., M. Nakazaro, S. Hashiguchi, K. Dezaki, M. S. Mondal, H. Hosoda, M. Kojima, K. Kangawa, T. Arima, H. Matsuo, et al. "Ghrelin Is Present in Pancreatic Alpha-Cells of Humans and Rats and Stimulates Insulin Secretion." *Diabetes* 51 (2002): 124–29.

Deponti, D., et al. "The Low Affinity Receptor for Neurotrophins p75NTR Plays a Key Role for Satellite Cell Function in Muscle Repair Acting via RhoA." *Cell* 20 (2009): 3620–27.

Dhillo, W. S., C. J. Small, S. A. Stanley, P. H. Jethwa, L. J. Seal, K. G. Murphy, M. A. Ghatei, and S. R. Bloom. "Hypothalamic Interactions between Neuropeptide Y, Agouti-Related Protein, Cocaine- and Amphetamine-Regulated Transcript and Alpha-Melanocyte-Stimulating Hormone in Vitro in Male Rats." *Journal of Neuroendocrinology* 14 (2002): 725–30.

Doherty, T. J. "Invited Review: Aging and Sarcopenia." *J. Appl Physiol* 95, no. 4 (2003): 1717–27.

Drewnowski, A., D. D. Krahn, M. A. Demitrack, K. Nairn, and B. A. Gosnell. "Taste Responses and Preferences for Sweet High-Fat Foods:

Evidence for Opioid Involvement." *Physiology and Behavior* 51 (1992): 371–79.

Dwivedi, Y. "Brain-Derived Neurotrophic Factor: Role in Depression and Suicide." *Neuropsychiatr. Dis. Treat.* 5 (2009): 433–49.

El-Khoury, A. E., N. K. Kukagawa, M. Sanchez, R. H. Tsay, R. E. Gleason, T. E. Chapman, and V. R. Young. "The 24-h Pattern and Rate of Leucine Oxidation, with Particular Reference to Tracer Estimates of Leucine Requirements in Healthy Adults." *Am. J. Clin. Nutr.* 59 (1994): 1012–20.

Ellacott, K. L., and R. D. Cone. "The Central Melanocortin System and the Integration of Short- and Long-Term Regulators of Energy Homeostasis." *Recent Progress in Hormone Research* 59 (2004): 395–408.

FAO/WHO/UNU. 1985. "Energy and Protein Requirements. Report of Joint FAO/WHO/UNU Expert Consultation." *WHO Tech. Rep. Sev.* 724 (1985): 1–206.

Fatemi, S. H. *Reelin Glycoprotein: Structure, Biology and Roles in Health and Disease.* Berlin: Springer, 2008.

Fernstrom, J. D., and R. J. Wurtman. "Brain Serotonin Content: Physiological Regulation by Plasma Neutral Amino Acids." Science 178 (1972): 414–16.

Fitts, R. H., and J. J. Widrick. "Muscle Mechanics: Adaptations with Exercise Training." *Exerc. Sport Sci. Rev.* 24 (1996): 427–73.

Floyd, J. C., S. S. Fajans, J. W. Conn, R. F. Knopl, and J. Rull. "Stimulation of Insulin Secretion by Amino Acids." *J. Clin. Invest.* 45 (1966): 1487–502.

Fornstrom, M. H., and J. D. Fernstrom. "Brain Tryptophan Concentrations and Scrotonin Synthesis Remain Responsive to Food Consumption after the Ingestion of Sequential Meals." *Am. J. Clin. Nutr.* 61 (1995): 312–19.

Friedl, K. E., R. J. Moore, R. W. Hoyt, L. J. Marchitelli, L. E. Martinez-Lopez, and E. W. Askew. "Endocrine Markers of Semistarvation in Healthy Lean Men in a Multistressor Environment." *J Appl Physiol.* 88, no. 5 (2000): 1820–30.

Fulton, S., B. Woodside, and P. Shizgal. "Modulation of Brain Reward Circuitry by Leptin." *Science* 287 (2000): 125–28.

Fulton, S., B. Woodside, and P. Shizgal. "Modulation of Brain Reward Circuitry by Leptin." *Science* 287 (2000): 125–28.

Garlick, P. J. "The Role of Leucine in the Regulation of Protein Metabolism." *J. Nutr.* 135, no. 6 (2005): S1553–56.

Gautsch, T. A., J. C. Anthony, S. R. Kimball, G. L. Paul, D. K. Layman, and L. S. Jefferson. "Availability of cIF4E Regulates Skeletal Muscle Protein Synthesis during Recovery from Exercise." *Am. J. Physiol. Cell Physiol.* 274 (1998): C406–14.

Ghiyath Shayeb, A., and S. Bhattacharya. "Review: Male Obesity and Reproductive Potential." *British Journal of Diabetes and Vascular Disease* 9, no. 1 (2009): 7–12.

Gibbs, J., R. C. Young, and G. P. Smith. "Cholecystokinin Decreases Food Intake in Rats." *Journal of Comparative Physiology and Psychology* 84 (1973): 488–95.

Gordon, T. "The Role of Neurotrophic Factors in Nerve Regeneration." *Neurosurg. Focus* 26 (2009): E3.

Grand, T. I. "Body Weight: Its Relation to Tissue Composition, Segment Distribution and Motor Function: I. Interspecific Comparisons." *Am. Jour. Phys. Anthrop.* 47 (1977): 241–48.

Griesbeck, O., A. S. Parsadanian, M. Sendtner, and H. Thoenen. "Expression of Neurotrophins in Skeletal Muscle: Quantitative Comparison and Significance of Motorneuron Survival and Maintenance of Function." *J. Neurosci. Res.* 42 (1995): 21–33.

Hagan, M. M., E. Castaneda, I. C. Sumaya, S. M. Fleming, J. Galloway, and D. E. Moss. "The Effect of Hypothalamic Peptide YY on Hippocampal Acetylcholine Release in Vivo: Implications for Limbic Function in Binge-Eating Behavior." *Brain Research* 805 (1998): 20–28.

Hagan, M. M., P. A. Rushing, S. C. Benoit, S. C. Woods, and R. J. Seeley. "Opioid Receptor Involvement in the Effect of AgRP (83-132) on Food Intake and Food Selection." *American Journal of Physiology Regulatory, Integrative and Comparative Physiology* 280 (2001): R814–21.

Hakansson, M. L., H. Brown, N. Ghilardi, R. C. Skoda, and B. Meister. "Leptin Receptor Immunoreactivity in Chemically Defined Target

Neurons of the Hypothalamus." *Journal of Neuroscience* 18 (1998): 559–72.

Hannan D. "Free Radical Theory of Aging: Role of Free Radicals in the Origination and Evolution of Life, Aging and Disease Process." In *Biology of Aging,* edited by J. Johnson, R. Walford, D. Hannan, and J. Miguel, 3–50. New York: Liss, 1986.

Hasten, D. L., J. Pak-Loduca, K. A. Obert, and K. E. Yarasheski. "Resistance Exercise Acutely Increases MHC and Mixed Muscle Protein Synthesis Rates in 78–84 and 23–32 Yr Olds." *Am. J. Physiol Endocrinol Metab.* 278, no. 4 (2000): 5620–26.

Henneman, E. "The Size Principle: A Deterministic Output Emerges from a Set of Probabilistic Connections." *Journal of Experimental Biology* 115 (1985): 105–12.

Hermann, C., R. Goke, G. Richter, H. C. Fehmann, R. Arnold, and B. Goke. "Glucagon-like Peptide-1 and Glucose-Dependent Insulin-Releasing Polypeptide Plasma Levels in Response to Nutrients." *British Journal of Pharmacology* 93 (1995): 79–84.

Heymsfield, S. B., A. S. Greenber, K. Fujioka, R. M. Dixon, R. Kushner, T. Hunt, J. A. Lubina, J. Patane, B. Self, P. Hunt, and M. McCamish. "Recombinant Leptin for Weight Loss in Obese and Lean Adults: A Randomized, Controlled, Dose-Escalation Trial." *Journal of the American Medical Association* 282 (1999): 1568–75.

Highfield, R. "Brain Scans Could Reveal Mental Strength." *Science,* October 18, 2007.

Hirsch, J., L. C. Hudgin, R. L. Leibel, and M. Rosenbaum. "Diet Composition and Energy Balance in Humans." *Am. J. Clin. Nutr.* 67 (1998): S551–55.

Holst, J. J. "Glucagon-like Peptide 1 (GLP-1): An Intestinal Hormone, Signaling Nutritional Abundance, with an Unusual Therapeutic Potential." *Trends in Endocrinology and Metabolism* 10 (1999): 229–35.

Holst, J. J. "Treatment of Type 2 Diabetes Mellitus with Agonists of the GLP-1 Receptor or DPP-IV Inhibitors." *Expert Opinion on Emerging Drugs* 9 (2004): 155–166.

Hotta, K., T. Funahashi, N. L. Bodkin, H. K. Ormeyer, Y. Rita, B. C. Hansen, and Y. Matsuzawa. "Circulating Concentrations of the Adipocyte Protein Adiponectin Are Decreased in Parallel with Reduced Insulin Sensitivity during the Progression to Type 2 Diabetes in Rhesus Monkeys." *Diabetes* 50 (2001): 1126–33.

Howell, F. C. "Recent Advances in Human Evolutionary Studies." *Quart. Rev. Biol.* 42 (1967): 471–513.

Hsich, R. H., J. H. Hou, H. S. Hsu, and Y. H. Wei. "Age-Dependent Respiratory Function Decline and DNA Deletions in Human Muscle Mitochondria." *Biochem. Mol. Biol. Int.* 32 (1994): 1009–22.

Huang, E. J., and L. F. Reichardt. "Neurotropins: Roles in Neuronal Development and Function." *Annu. Rev. Neurosci.* 24 (2001): 677–736.

Hunt, J. V., R. T. Dean, and S. P. Wolff. "Hydroxyl Radical Production and Autoxidative Glycosylation: Glucose Autoxidation as the Cause of Protein Damage in the Experimental Glycation Model of Diabetes Mellitus and Ageing." *Biochem. J.* 256 (1988): 205–12.

Jin, X., et al. "Opposite Roles of MRF4 and MyoD in Cell Proliferation and Mygenic Differentiation." *Biochem. Biophys. Res. Commun.* 364 (2007): 476–82.

Jolly, C. J. "The Seed-Eaters: A New Model of Hominid Differentiation Based on a Baboon Analogy." *Royal Anthropology Institute of Great Britain and Ireland: Man, New Series,* 5, no. 1 (1970): 5–26.

Jostarndt-Fogen, K., A. Puntschart, H. Hoppeler, and R. Billeter. "Fibre-Type Specific Expression of Fast and Slow Essential Myosin Light Chain mRNAs in Trained Human Skeletal Muscles." *Acta. Physiol. Scand.* 164 (1998): 299–308.

Jubrias, S. A., P. C. Esselman, L. B. Price, M. E. Cress, and K. E. Conley. "Large Energetic Adaptations of Elderly Muscle to Resistance and Endurance Training." *J. Appl Physiol.* 90, no. 5 (2001): 1663–70.

Kablar, B., and A. C. Belliveau. "Presence of Neurotrophic Factors in Skeletal Muscle Correlates with Survival of Spinal Cord Motor Neurons." *Dev. Dyn.* 234 (2005): 659–60.

Kaplan, A. S., R. S. Levitan, Z. Yilmaz, C. Davis, S. Tharmalingam, and J. L. Kennedy. "A DRD4/BDNF Gene-Gene Interaction Associated with Maximum BMI in Women with Bulimia Nervosa." *Int. J. Eat. Disord.* 41, no. 1 (2008): 22–28.

Karlsson J. "Exercise, Muscle Metabolism and the Antioxidant Defense." *World Rev. Nutr. Diet.* 82 (1997): 81–100.

Kasturi, S. S., J. Tannir, and R. E. Brannigan. "The Metabolic Syndrome and Male Infertility." *J Androl.* 29, no. 3 (2008): 251–59.

Kermani, P., and B. Hempstead. "Brain-Derived Neurotrophic Factor: A Newly Described Mediator of Angiogenesis." *Trends Cardiovasc. Med.* 17 (2007): 140–143.

Kerschensteiner, M., et al. "Activated Human T Cells, B Cells, and monocytes Produce Brain-Derived Neurotrophic Factor in Vitro and in Inflammatory Brain Lesions: A Neurtroprotective Role of Inflammation?" *J. Exp. Med.* 189 (1999): 865–870.

Kimball, S. R., and L. S. Jefferson. "Regulation of Protein Synthesis by Branched-Chain Amino Acids." *Curr. Opin. Clin. Nutr. Metab. Care* 4 (2001): 39–43.

Kissileff, H. R., J. C. Carretta, A. Geliebter, and F. X. Pi-Sunyer. "Cholecystokinin and Stomach Distension Combine to Reduce Food Intake in Humans." *American Journal of Physiology—Regulatory, Integrative and Comparative Physiology* 285 (2003): R992–98.

Koopman, R., and L. J. van Loon. "Aging, Exercise, and Muscle Protein Metabolism." *J Appl Physiol.* 106 (2009): 2040–48.

Krebs, M., M. Krssak, E. Bemroider, C. Anderwald, A. Brehm, M. Meyerspeer, P. Nowotny, E. Roth, W. Waldhausl, and M. Roden. "Mechanism of Amino Acid-Induced Skeletal Muscle Insulin Resistance in Humans." *Diabetes* 51 (2002): 599–605.

Kreymann, B., G. Williams, M. A. Ghatei, and S. R. Blood. "Glucagon-Like Peptide-1 7-36: A Physiological Incretin in Man." *Lancet* 2 (1987): 1300–1304.

Kristensen, P., M. E. Judge, L. Thim, U. Ribel, K. N. Christjarsen, B. S. Wulff, J. T. Clausen, P. B. Jensen, O. D. Madsen, N. Vrang, P. J. Larsen, and S. Hastrup. "Hypothalamic CART Is a New Anorectic Peptide Regulated by Leptin." *Nature* 393 (1998): 72–76.

Krude, H., H. Biebermann, W. Luck, R. Horn, G. Brabant, and A. Gruters. "Severe Early-Onset Obesity, Adrenal Insufficiency and Red Hair Pigmentation Caused by POMC Mutations in Humans." *Nature Genetics* 19 (1998): 155–57.

Laaksonen, D. E., L. Niskanen, K. Punnonen, K. Nyyssönen, T.P. Tuomainen, V.P. Valkonen, and J. T. Salonen. "The Metabolic Syndrome and Smoking in Relation to Hypogonadism in Middle-Aged Men: A Prospective Cohort Study." *Journal of Clinical Endocrinology and Metabolism* 90, no. 2 (2005): 712–19.

Laaksonen, D. E., L. Niskanen, K. Punnonen, K. Nyyssönen, T. P. Tuomainen, V. P. Valkonen, R. Salonen, and J. T. Salonen. "Testosterone and Sex Hormone-Binding Globulin Predict the Metabolic Syndrome and Diabetes in Middle-Aged Men." *Diabetes Care* 27, no. 5 (2004): 1036–41.

Lacaille, B., P. Julien, Y. Deshaies, C. Lavigne, L. D. Brun, and H. Jacques. "Responses of Plasma Lipoproteins and Sex Hormones to the Consumption of Lean Fish Incorporated in a Prudent-Type Diet in Normolipidemic Men." *J Am Coll Nutr.* 19, no. 6 (2000): 745–53.

Lancaster, C. S., et al. "The Evolution of Hunting." In *Man the Hunter,* edited by R. B. Lee and I. DeVore. Chicago: Aldine, 1968.

Larsson, L., G. Grimby, and J. Karlsson. "Muscle Strength and Speed of Movement in Relation to Age and Muscle Morphology." *J. Appl. Physiol.* 46 (1979): 451–56.

Layman, D. K. "Role of Leucine in Protein Metabolism during Exercise and Recovery." *Can. J. Appl. Physiol.* 27 (2002): 592–608.

———. "The Role of Leucine in Weight Loss Diets and Glucose Homeostasis." *J. Nutr.* 133 (2003): S261–67.

Layman, D. K., and J. I. Baum. "Dietary Protein Impact on Glycemic Control during Weight Loss: The American Society for Nutritional Sciences." *J Nutr.* 134 (2004): S968S–73.

————. "The Emerging Role of Dairy Proteins and Bioactive Peptides in Nutrition and Health: The American Society for Nutritional Sciences." *J. Nutr.* 134 (2004): S968–73.

Layman, D. K., E. M. Evans, D. Erickson, J. Seyler, J. Weber, O. Bagshaw, A. Griel, A. Psota, P. Kris-Etherton. "A Moderate Protein Diet Produces Sustained Weight Loss and Long-Term Changes in Body Composition and Blood Lipids in Obese Adults." *J. Nutr.* 139, no. 3 (2009): 514–21.

Layman, D. K., and D. A. Walker. "Potential Importance of Leucine in Treatment of Obesity and the Metabolic Syndrome." *J. Nutr.* 136, no. 1 (2006): S319–23.

Layman, D. K., R. A. Boileau, D. J. Erickson, J. E. Painter, H. Shiue, C. Sather, and D. D. Christou. "A Reduced Ratio of Dietary Carbohydrate to Protein Improves Body Composition and Blood Lipid Profiles during Weight Loss in Men." *J. Nutr.* 133 (2003): 411–17.

Layman, D. K., H. Shiue, C. Sather, D. J. Erickson, and J. Baum. "Increased Dietary Protein Modifies Glucose and Insulin Homeostasis in Adult Women during Weight Loss." *J. Nutr.* 133 (2003): 405–10.

Lee, C. K., R. C. Klopp, R. Weindruch, and T. A. Prolla. "Gene Expression Profile of Aging and Its Retardation by Calorie Restriction." *Science* 285 (1999): 1390–3.

Lee, H. M., V. Udupi, E. W. Englander, S. Rajaraman, R. J. Coffee Jr., and G. H. Greeley. "Stimulatory Actions of Insulin-Like Growth Factor-1 and Transforming Growth Factor-Alpha on Intestinal Neurotensin and Peptide YY." *Endocrinology* 140 (1999): 4065–69.

Leewenburgh, C., R. Fiebig, R. Chandwancy, and L. L. Ji. "Aging and Exercise Training in Skeletal Muscle: Responses of Glutathione and Antioxidant Enzyme Systems." *Am. J. Physiol.* 267 (1994): R439–45.

Lemon, P. W. R. "Beyond the Zone: Protein Needs of Active Individuals." *J. Am. Coll. Nutr.* 19 (2000): S513–21.

Lexell, J. "Human Aging, Muscle Mass, and Fiber Type Composition." *J. Gerontol A. Biol Sci. Med. Sci.* 50A (1995): 11–16.

Lexell, J., and D. Downham. "What Is the Effect of Ageing on Type 2 Muscle Fibres?" *J. Neurol. Sci.* 107 (1992): 250–1.

Li, C., E. S. Ford, B. Li, W. H. Giles, and S. Liu. "Association of Testosterone and Sex Hormone-Binding Globulin with Metabolic Syndrome and Insulin Resistance in Men." *Diabetes Care* 33, no. 7 (2010): 1618–24.

Liddle, R. A., I. D. Goldfine, M. S. Rosen, R. A. Taplitz, and J. A. Williams. "Cholecystokinin Bioactivity in Human Plasma: Molecular Forms, Responses to Feeding, and Relationship to Gallbladder Contraction." *Journal of Clinical Investigation* 75 (1985): 1144–52.

Lin, L., R. Martin, A. O. Schaffhauser, and D. A. York. "Acute Changes in the Response to Peripheral Leptin with Alteration in the Diet Composition." *American Journal of Physiology: Regulatory, Integrative and Comparative Physiology* 280 (2001): R504–9.

Lipton, B. R., and E. Schultz. "Developmental Fate of Skeletal Muscle Satellite Cells." *Science* 205 (1979): 1292–94.

Livingston, F. B. "Reconstructing Man's Pliocene Pongid Ancestor." *Am. Anthrop.* 64 (1962): 301–5.

Livingstone, C., and M. Collison. "Sex Steroids and Insulin Resistance." *Clinical Science* 102 (2002): 151–66.

Lord, G. M., G. Matarese, J. K. Howard, R. J. Baker, S. R. Bloom, and R. I. Lechler. "Leptin Modulates the T-Cell Immune Response and Reverses Starvation-Induced Immunosuppression." *Nature* 394 (1998): 897–901.

Maina, G., G. Rosso, R. Zanardini, F. Bogetto, M. Gennarelli, and L. Boochio-Chiavetto. "Serum Levels of Brain-Derived Neurotrophic Factor in Drug-Native Obsessive-Compulsive Patients: A Case-Control Study." *J. Affect. Disord.* 122, no. 1–2 (2009): 174–78.

Makimura, H., T. M. Mizuno, J. W. Mastaitis, R. Agami, and C. V. Mobbs. "Reducing Hypothalamic AGRP by RNA Interference Increases Metabolic Rate and Decreases Body Weight without Influencing Food Intake." *BMC Neuroscience* 3 (2002): 18.

Makrdies, L., J. G. Heigenhauser, N. McCartney, and N. L. Jones. "Maximal Short-Term Exercise Capacity in Healthy Subjects Aged 13–70 Years." *Clin. Sci. Lond.* 69 (1996): 197–205.

Mandel, A. L., H. Ozdener, and V. Utermohlen. "Identification of Pro- and Mature Brain-Derived Neurotrophic Factor in Human Saliva." *Arch. Oral. Biol.* 54, no. 7 (2009): 689–95.

Marx, J. O., W. J. Kraemer, B. C. Nindl, and L. Larsson. "Effects of Aging on Human Skeletal Muscle Myosin Heavy-Chain mRNA Content and Protein Isoform Expression." *J Gerontol A. Biol. Sci. Med. Sci.* 57, no. 6 (2002): B232–38.

Mattson. M. "The Need for Controlled Studies of the Effects of Meal Frequency on Health." *Lancet* 365 (2005): 1978–80.

Mattson, M. P. "Glutamate and Neurotrophic Factors in Neuronal Plasticity and Disease." *Annals of the New York Academy of Sciences* 1144 (2008): 97–90.

Menendez, J. A., and D. M. Atrens. "Insulin and the Paraventricular Hypothalamus: Modulation of Energy Balance." *Brain Research* 555 (1991): 193–201.

Mercader, J. M., F. Fernández-Aranda, M. Gratacòs, M. Ribasés, A. Badia, C. Villarejo, R. Solano, J. R. González, J. Vallejo, and X. Estivill. "Blood Levels of Brain-Derived Neurotrophic Factor Correlate with Several Psychopathological Symptoms in Anorexia Nervosa Patients." *Neuropsychobiology* 56, no. 4 (2007): 185–90.

Miguel, J., and J. Fleming. "Theoretical and Experimental Support for an 'Oxygen Radical Mitochondrial Injury' Hypothesis of Cell Aging." In *Biology of Aging,* edited by J. Johnson, R. Walford, D. Harman, and J. Miquel, 51–76. New York: Liss, 1993.

Millward, D. J., D. K. Layman, D. Tome, and G. Schaafsma. "Protein Quality Assessment: Impact of Expanding Understanding of Protein and Amino Acid Needs for Optimal Health." *Am. J. Clinical Nutrition* 87, no. 5 (2008): S1576–81.

Moncada, S., and E. A. Higgs. "Molecular Mechanisms and Therapeutic Strategies Related to Nitric Oxide." *FASEB J.* 9 (1995): 1319–30.

Mousavi, K., and B. J. Jasmin. "BDNF Is Expressed in Skeletal Muscle Satellite Cells and Inhibits Myogenic Differentiation. *J. Neurosci.* 26 (2006): 5739–49.

Mousavi, K., D. J. Parry, and B. J. Jasmin. "BDNF Rescues Myosin Heavy Chain IIB Muscle Fibers after Neonatal Nerve Injury." *Am. J. Physiol. Cell Physiol.* 287 (2004): C22–29.

Naslund, E., B. Barkeling, N. King, M. Gutnaik, J. E. Blundell, J. J. Holst, S. Rossner, and P. M. Hellstrom. "Energy Intake and Appetite Are Suppressed by Glucagon-Like Peptide-1 (GLP-1) in Obese Men." *International Journal of Obesity and Related Metabolic Disorders* 23 (1999): 304–11.

Naslund, E., J. Bogefors, S. Skogar, P. Gryback, H. Jacobsson, J. J. Holst, and P. M. Hellstrom. "GLP-1 Slows Solid Gastric Emptying and Inhibits Insulin, Glucagon, and PYY Release in Humans." *American Journal of Physiology: Regulatory, Integrative and Comparative Physiology* 277 (1999): R910–16.

Nauck, M. A., N. Kleine, C. Orskov, J. J. Holst, B. Willms, and W. Creutzfeldt. "Normalization of Fasting Hyperglycaemia by Exogenous Glucagon-Like Peptide 1 (7-36 Amide) in Type 2 (Non-Insulin-Dependent) Diabetic Patients." *Diabetologia* 36 (1993): 741–44.

Nicolaidis, S., and N. Rowland. "Metering of Intravenous versus Oral Nutrients and Regulation of Energy Balance." *American Journal of Physiology* 231 (1976): 661–68.

Norton, L. E., and D. K. Layman. "Leucine Regulates Translation Initiation of Protein Synthesis in Skeletal Muscle after Exercise." *J. Nutr.* 136, no. 2 (2006): S533–37.

Obici, S., Z. Feng, G. Karkanias, D. G. Baskin, and L. Rossetti. "Decreasing Hypothalamic Insulin Receptors Causes Hyperphagia and Insulin Resistance in Rats." *Nature Neuroscience* 5 (2002): 566–72.

Oppenheimer, A. "Tool Use and Crowded Teeth in Australopithecinae." *Curr. Anthrop.* 5 (1964): 419–21.

Otto, B., U. Cuntz, E. Fruehauf, R. Wawarta, C. Folwaczmy, R. L. Riepl, M. L. Heiman, P. Lehnert, M. Fichter, and M. Tschop. "Weight Gain Decreases Elevated Plasma Ghrelin Concentrations of Patients with Anorexia Nervosa." *European Journal of Endocrinology* 145 (2001): 669–73.

Pacy, P. J., G. M. Price, D. Halliday, M. R. Quevedo, and D. J. Millward. "Nitrogen Homeostasis in Man: The Diurnal Responses of Protein Synthesis and Degradation and Amino Acid Oxidation to Diets with Increasing Protein Intakes." *Clin. Sci.* 86 (1994): 103–18.

Paddon-Jones, D., M. Sheffield-Moore, X. J. Zhang, E. Volpi, S. E. Wolf, A. Aarsland, A. A. Ferrando, and R. R. Wolfe. "Amino Acid Ingestion Improves Muscle Protein Synthesis in the Young and Elderly." *Am. J. Physiol Endocrinol. Metab.* 286, no. 3 (2004): E321–28.

Paddon-Jones, D., E. Westman, R. D. Mattes, R. R. Wolfe, A. Astrup, and M. Westerterp-Phantenga. "Protein, Weight Management, and Satiety." *Am. J. Clinical Nutrition* 87, no. 5 (2008): S1558–61.

Pasquali, R., F. Casimirri, R. De Iasio, P. Mesini, S. Boschi, R. Chierici, R. Flamia, M. Biscotti, and V. Vicennati. "Insulin Regulates Testosterone and Sex Hormone-Binding Globulin Concentrations in Adult Normal Weight and Obese Men." *Journal of Clinical Endocrinology and Metabolism* 80 (1995): 654–58.

Pederson-Bjergaard, U., U. Host, H. Kelback, S. Schifter, J. F. Rehfeld, J. Faber, and N. J. Christensen. "Influence of Meal Composition of Postprandial Peripheral Plasma Concentrations of Vasoactive Peptides in Man." *Scandinavian Journal of Clinical and Laboratory Investigation* 56 (1996): 497–503.

Pillbeam, D. R., and E. L. Simons. "Some Problems of Hominid Classification." *Am. Sci.* 53 (1965): 237–59.

Pitteloud, N., M. Hardin, A. A. Dwyer, E. Valassi, M. Yialamas, D. Elahi, and F. J. Hayes. "Increasing Insulin Resistance Is Associated with a Decrease in Leydig Cell Testosterone Secretion in Men." *Journal of Clinical Endocrinology and Metabolism* 90, no. 5 (2005): 2636–41.

Polonsky, K. S., B. D. Given, and E. Van Cauter. "Twenty-Four Hour Profiles and Pulsatile Patterns of Insulin Secretion in Normal and Obese Subjects." *Journal of Clinical Investigation* 81 (1988): 442–48.

Porte, D., Jr., D. G. Baskin, and M. W. Schwartz. "Leptin and Insulin Action in the Central Nervous System." *Nutritional Reviews* 60 (2002): S20–29.

Putman, C. T., N. L. Jones, L. C. Lands, T. M. Blagg, M. G. Hollidge-Horvat, and C. J. Heigenhauser. "Skeletal Muscle Pyruvate Dehydrogenase Activity during Maximal Exercise in Humans." *Am J. Physiol.* 269, no. 32 (1995): E458–68.

Reavens, G. M. "Role of Insulin Resistance in Human Disease (Syndrome X): An Expanded Definition." *Annu. Rev. Mod.* 44 (1993): 121–131.

Reddypalli, S., K. Roll, H. K. Lee, M. Lundell, E. Barea-Rodriguez, and E. F. Wheeler. "p75NTR-Mediated Signaling Promotes the Survival of Myoblasts and Influences Muscle Strength." *J. Cell. Physiol.* 204 (2005): 810–29.

Reeds, P. J., D. G. Burrin, T. A. Davis, and B. Stoll. "Amino Acid Metabolism and the Energetic of Growth." *Arch. Anim. Nutr.* 51 (1998): 187–97.

Rennie, M. J, and K. D. Tipton. "Protein and Amino Acid Metabolism during and after Exercise and the Effects of Nutrition." *Annu. Rev. Nutr.* 20 (2000): 457–83.

Reynolds, G. "Phys Ed: The Benefits of Exercising Before Breakfast." http://well.blogs.nytimes.com/2010/12/15/phys-ed-the-benefits-of-exercising-before-breakfast/?ref=gretchenreynolds, December 15, 2010.

Rios, M., G. Fan, C. Fekete, J. Kelly, B. Bates, R. Kuehn, R. M. Lechan, and R. Jaenisch. "Conditional Deletion of Brain-Derived Neurotrophic Factor in the Postnatal Brain Leads to Obesity and Hyperactivity." *Mol. Endocrinol.* 15 (2001): 1748–57.

Roubenoff, R. "Sarcopenia: Effects on Body Composition and Function." *J. Gerontol. A. Biol. Sci. Med. Sci.* 58, no. 11 (2003): M1012–17.

Ruderman, N. B. "Muscle Amino Acid Metabolism and Gluconcogenesis." *Ann. Rev. Med.* 26 (1975): 245–58.

Russo-Neustadt, A. A., R. C. Beard, Y. M. Huang, and C. W. Cotman. "Physical Activity and Antidepressant Treatment Potentiate the Expression of Specific Brain-Derived Neutotropic Factor Transcripts in the Rat Hippocampus." *Neuroscience* 101, no. 2 (2000): 305–12.

Sale, D. G. "Influence of Exercise and Training on Motor Unit Activation." *Exercise and Sports Science Reviews* 15 (1987): 95–151.

Saper, C. B., T. C. Chou, and J. K. Elmquist. "The Need to Feed: Homeostatic and Hedonic Control of Eating." *Neuron* 36 (2002): 199–211.

Seale, P., L. A. Sabourin, A. Girgis-Gabardo, A. Mansouri, P. Gruss, and M. A. Rudnicki. "Pax7 Is Required for the Specification of Myogenic Satellite Cells." *Cell* 102 (2000): 777–86.

Seidl, K., C. Erck, and A. Buchberger. "Evidence for Participation of Nerve Growth Factor and Its Low-Affinity Receptor in the Regulation of the Myogenic Program." *J. Cell. Physiol.* 176 (1998): 10–21.

Shipman, P., and A. Walker. "The Costs of Becoming a Predator." *Journal of Human Evolution* 18 (1969): 373–392.

Short, K. R., J. L. Vittone, M. L. Bigelow, D. N. Proctor, and K. S. Nair. "Age and Aerobic Exercise Training Effects on Whole Body and Muscle Protein Metabolism." *Am. J. Physiol. Endocrinol. Metab.* 286, no. 1 (2004): E92–101.

Simons, E. L. "The Hunt for Darwin's Third Ape." *Med. Opinion Rev.* (November 1965): 74–81.

Skov, A. R., S. Toubro, B. Ronn, L. Holm, and A. Astrup. "Randomized Trial on Protein vs. Carbohydrate in Ad Libitum Fat Reduced Diet for the Treatment of Obesity." *Int. J. Obes.* 23 (1999): 528–36.

Staron, R. S., E. S. Malicky, M. J. Leonardi, et al. "Muscle Hypertrophy and Fast Fiber Type Conversions in Heavy Resistance-Trained Women." *Eur. J. Appl. Physiol. Occup. Physiol.* 60 (1990): 71–79.

Stellar, E. "The Physiology of Motivation." *Psychological Review* 101 (1954): 301–11.

Stratford, T. R., and A. E. Kelley. "Evidence of a Functional Relationship between the Nucleus Accumbens Shell and Lateral Hypothalamus Subserving the Control of Feeding Behavior." *Journal of Neuroscience* 19 (1999): 11040–48.

Strobel, A., T. Issad, L. Camoin, M. Ozata, and A. D. Strosberg. "A Leptin Missense Mutation Associated with Hypogonadism and Morbid Obesity." *Nature Genetics* 18 (1998): 213–15.

Sun, Y., P. Wang, H. Zheng, and R. G. Smith. "Ghrelin Stimulation of Growth Hormone Release and Appetite Is Mediated through the Growth Hormone Secretagogue Receptor." *PNAS* 101 (2004): 4679–84.

Svanberg, E., L. S. Jefferson, K. Lundhold, and S. R. Kimball. "Postprandial Stimulation of Muscle Protein Synthesis Is Independent of Changes in Insulin." *Endocrinology and Metabolism* 272, no. 5 (1997): E841–47.

Szczypka, M. S., K. Kwok, M. D. Brot, B. T. Marck, A. M. Matsumoto, B. A. Donahue, and R. D. Palmiter. "Dopamine Production in the Caudate Putamen Restores Feeding in Dopamine-Deficient Mice." *Neuron* 30 (2001): 819–28.

Taylor, S. M. "Electroconvulsive Therapy, Brain-Derived Neurotrophic Factor, and Possible Neurorestorative Benefit of the Clinical Application of Electroconvulsive Therapy." *Journal of ECT* 24, no. 2 (2008): 160–65.

Tidball, J. G. "Inflammatory Processes in Muscle Injury and Repair." *Am. J. Physiol. Regul. Integr. Comp. Physiol.* 288 (2005): R345–53.

Tiidus, P. M. "Radical Species in Inflammation and Overtraining." *Can. J. Physiol. Pharmacol.* 76, no. 5 (1998): 533–38.

Traish, A. M., F. Saad, and A. Guay. "The Dark Side of Testosterone Deficiency: II. Type 2 Diabetes and Insulin Resistance." *J. Androl.* 30, no. 1 (2009): 23–32.

Turrens, J. F., J. Lariccia, and M. G. Nair. "Resveratrol Has No Effect on Lipoprotein Profile and Does Not Prevent Peroxidation of Serum Lipids in Normal Rats." *Free Radic. Res.* 27 (1997): 557–62.

van Dam, E. W., J. M. Dekker, E. G. Lentjes, F. P. Romijn, Y. M. Smulders, W. J. Post, J. A. Romijn, and H. M. Krans. "Steroids in Adult Men with Type 1 Diabetes: A Tendency to Hypogonadism." *Diabetes Care* 26, no. 6 (2003): 1812–18.

Van Proeyen, K., K. Szlufcik, H. Nielens, K. Pelgrim, L. Deldicque, M. Hesselink, P. P. Van Veldhoven, and P. Hespel. "Training in the Fasted State Improves Glucose Tolerance during Fat-Rich Diet." *J. Physiol.* 588, pt. 21 (2010): 4289–302.

Varga-Perez, H., A. Ting, R. Kee, C. Walton, et al. "Ventral Tegmental Area BDNF Induces an Opiate-Dependent-Like Reward State in Naïve Rates." *Science* 324, no. 5935 (2009): 1732–34.

Wagenmaker, A. J. M. "Muscle Amino Acid Metabolism at Rest and During Exercise: Role in Human Physiology and Metabolism." *Exerc. Sport Sci. Rev.* 26 (1998): 287–314.

Walker, A. "The Strength of Great Apes and the Speed of Humans." *Curr. Anthrop.* 50, no. 2 (2009).

Willer, C. J., E. K. Speliotes, R. J. Loos, et al. "Six New Loci Associated with Body Mass Index Highlight a Neuronal Influence on Body Weight Regulation." *Nat. Genat.* 41, no. 1 (2009): 24–34.

Wu, G., and S. M. Morris. "Arginine Metabolism: Nitric Oxide and Beyond." *Biochem. J.* 336 (1998): 1–17.

Wynne, K., S. Stanley, B. McGowan, and S. Bloom. "Appetite Control." *Journal of Endocrinology* 184 (2005): 291–318.

Xin, M. H., L. Hui, Y. F. Dang, T. De Hon, C. X. Zhang, Y. L. Zheng, D. C. Chen, T. R. Kosten, and X. Y. Zhang. "Decreased Serum BDNF Levels in Chronic Institutionalized Schizophrenia on Long-Term Treatment and Atypical Antipsychotics." *Prog. Neuropsychopharmacol. Biol. Psychiatry* 33, no. 8 (2009): 1508–12.

Xu, Y., B. Ku, L. Tie, H. Yao, W. Jiang, X. Ma, and X. Li. "Curcumin Reverses the Effects of Chronic Stress on Behavior, the HPA Axis, BDNF Expression and Phosphorylation of CREB." *Brain Research* 1122, no. 1 (2006): 56.

Yamada, K., and T. Nabeshima. "Brain-Derived Neurotrophic Factor/TrkB Signaling in Memory Processes." *J. Pharmacol. Sci.* 91, no. 4 (2003): 267–70.

Zigova, T., V. Pencea, S. J. Wiegand, and M. B. Luskin. "Intraventricular Administration of BDNF Increases the Number of Newly Generated Neurons in the Adult Olfactory Bulb." *Mol. Cell. Neurosci.* 11, no. 4 (1998): 234–45.

Zihlman, A. "Behavior and Human Evolution." In *Classification and Human Evolution*, edited by S. L. Washburn. Chicago: Aldine, 1963.

———. "The Evolution of Bipedal Walking in the Hominids." *Arch. Biol. (Liège)*, 75 (1964): S673–708.

———. "Locomotion as a Life History Character: The Contribution of Anatomy." *Journal of Human Evolution* 22 (1992): 315–325.

———. "Observations on the Strength of the Chimpanzee and Its Implications." *Journal of Mammalogy* 7 (1926): 1–9.

Zuccato, C., and E. Cattaneo. "Brain-Derived Neurotrophic Factor in Neurodegenerative Diseases." *Nat. Rev. Neurol.* 5, no. 6 (2009): 311–22.

Index

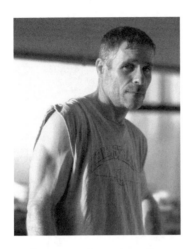

About the Author

Ori Hofmekler is a modern-day Renaissance man whose formative military experience prompted a lifelong interest in survival science. A graduate of the Bezalel Academy of Art and the Hebrew University in Jerusalem, where he received a degree in human science, Hofmekler is a world-renowned artist whose work has been featured in magazines worldwide. His art books of political satire have been published in the United States and Europe. As editor-in-chief of *Mind and Muscle Power* magazine, Hofmekler introduced his diet approach to the public to immediate acclaim from readers and professionals. His book *The Warrior Diet* was first published in 2002 in the United States, France, and Italy and has been featured in newspapers, magazines, and science journals. A new, revised edition was published in 2007. Hofmekler's 2006 book, *The Anti-Estrogenic Diet,* provides solutions to hormonal-disrupting chemicals in the environment, food, and water. His *Take No Prisoners* newsletter exposes fallacies in the areas of diet and fitness and presents the true facts about human survival in today's world. For more information about Hofmekler's nutritional and training protocols and to receive his newsletters and blogs, visit www.warriordiet.com or www.defensenutrition.com.